VINTAGE SECRETS

Hollywood Beauty

VINTAGE SECRETS

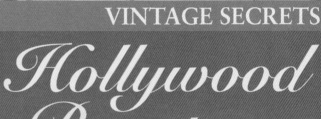

Hollywood Beauty

Laura Slater

Plexus, London

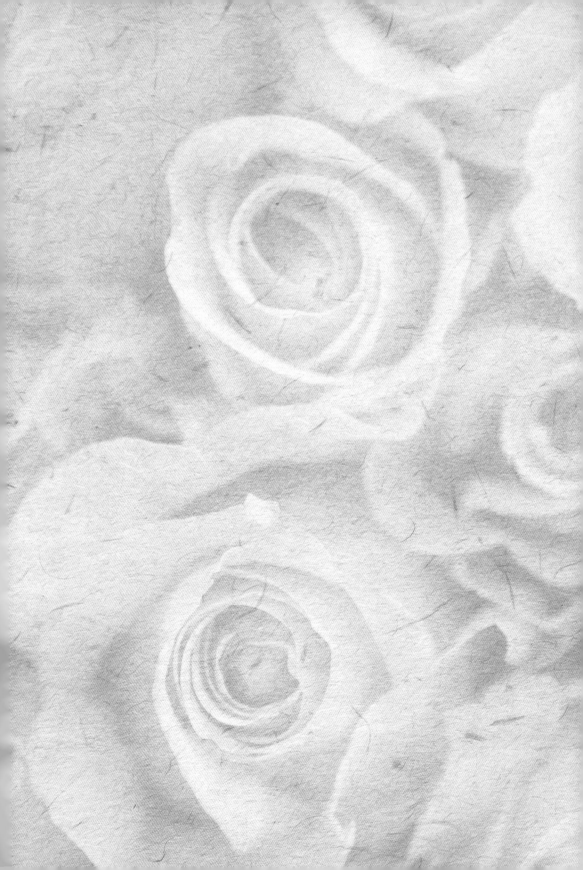

Contents

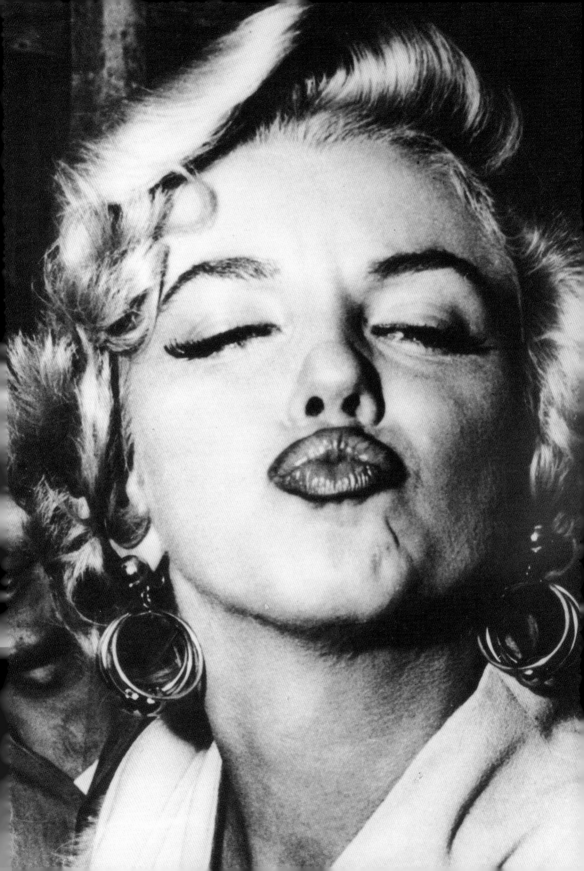

Introduction

Beauty on Screen

*'The lipstick and mascara were like clothes,
I saw that they improved my looks as much
as if I had put on a real gown.'*
– Marilyn Monroe

For a long time prior to the 1920s, makeup was the preserve of a 'certain sort' of woman. Actresses and prostitutes were, at one time, virtually indistinguishable. Instead of turning to bottled beauty, nicely brought-up girls relied on biting their lips and pinching their cheeks to create natural colour. That all changed with the rise of Hollywood. As films – and their stars – became more popular, so did the makeup worn by these beauties of the screen.

Initially – back in the plastic decade that was the 1920s – movie stars were obliged to resort to heavy makeup to have their features show up on screen at all. Out in the world, fans copied their style anyway. As movie cameras and lighting improved, however, screen makeup became lighter and fashion, still following Hollywood, embraced the natural look too. When Hollywood turned to red-lipped pin-ups to boost wartime morale, the world was awash with weekend Rita Hayworths – all dressed practically for workday duties, of course, and ready to 'do their bit'. The fifties saw a revival of the twenties artificial styles, perhaps in the elation of peace, while the sixties celebrated youth with pretty pastels and wide, baby-doll eyes.

Marilyn Monroe.

According to Max Factor and his successor Max, Jr. (who both kept detailed diaries of changing trends), fashions in beauty change roughly every five years and, during Hollywood's golden age, each new trend coincided with the rise of a new star. First there was lovely Mary Pickford, whose abundant golden curls made her America's sweetheart; she was followed by exotic beauty Gloria Swanson, who wore her dark hair short and slick, and then Mae Murray, whose tiny, bee-stung lips made her the envy of women everywhere.

The Dutch bobs worn by Colleen Moore and Louise Brooks were all the rage until tempestuous redhead Clara Bow took centre-stage, casting all others into the shade. But even It girl Clara eventually gave way to the WooWoo girls – whose leader Joan Crawford was simply all eyes and lips. Right up until her untimely death in 1937, it seemed Jean Harlow would rule forever . . . who knew it would take one Marilyn Monroe to resurrect her blonde bombshell style decades later?

'I know that one of the things
I should thank Hollywood for most is teaching
me how to put on the right kind of makeup.
My hat is off to Wally Westmore forever.'
– Dorothy Lamour

It was only really in the 1960s that fashion began influencing Hollywood, rather than the other way around. In 1967's *Two for the Road*, Audrey Hepburn is a walking advertisement for each of the decade's most far-out trends, via a dizzying 150 costume changes.

Today, of course, 'vintage' has become the most wonderfully eclectic kind of umbrella term – to be embraced in whichever manner you choose. We can even *mix* styles and eras – why not? Vintage style is all about cherry-picking looks and techniques from the past and incorporating them into your own life. How you wear them is entirely up to you – it's your style, after all.

So, whether you are a dedicated follower of forties fashion or prefer to flit from the twenties to the sixties on a daily basis, this book provides tips and tricks to guide you – direct from the most glamorous women of the silver screen and the pros who gave them a helping hand.

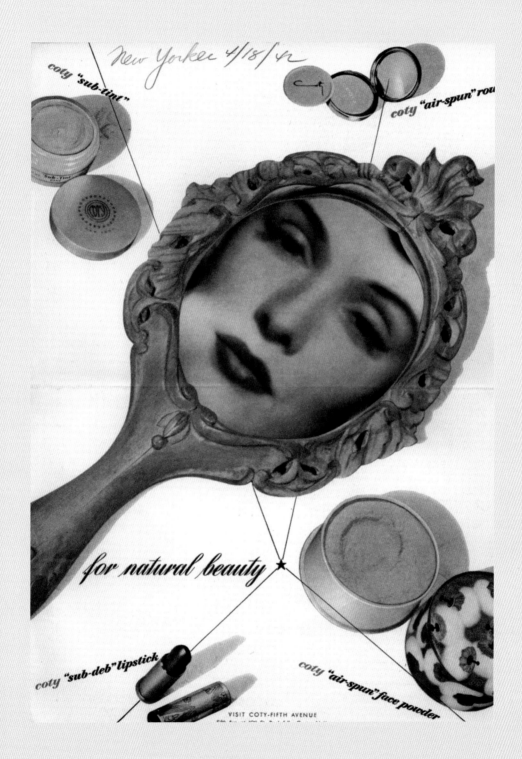

coty "sub-tint"

New Yorker 4/18/42

coty "air-spun" rou...

for natural beauty

coty "sub-deb" lipstick

coty "air-spun" face powder

VISIT COTY-FIFTH AVENUE

Makeup

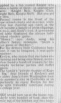
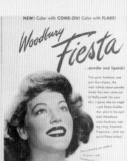
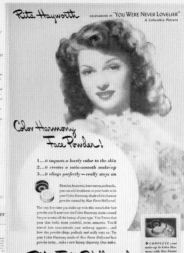
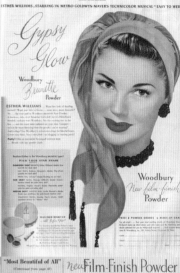
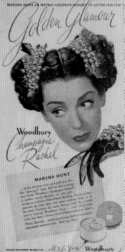
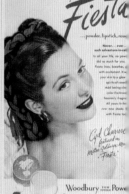

Preparing for Perfection

CHOOSING YOUR COLOUR SCHEME

'Those who rush out and haphazardly buy boxes
of this and bottles of that become – to borrow
Perc Westmore's word – makeup-a-holics.'
– Joan Crawford

Once upon a time, powder always meant white, with most girls striving for the ultra-pale look of the aristocracy. Then, in the twenties, a broader range of shades made it possible for women to match their makeup more closely to their own skin tone. In Hollywood, Max Factor brought in the concept of 'colour harmony'. Using the screen beauties he worked with as living examples, Max encouraged women to play to their strengths.

Sass-talking siren Mae West was well aware of the pitfalls of fighting what nature gave you: if you're naturally pale, dark makeup will only turn you orange; if you're darker skinned, wearing light makeup won't make you 'fair as a day in May'. Instead, you'll end up looking like 'a Hallowe'en goblin'. While subtle adjustments can be flattering (who doesn't suit the glow you get from tinted moisturiser in summer?), more drastic changes should be avoided at all costs.

Regardless of what's on trend, it's

'Makeup ought to look
as if it were nature's
own bloom upon you.'
– Mae West

important to stick with shades and products that suit you. You might adore the strong red lips of the 1940s, but if they make you look pale and drawn, they're honestly best avoided. So, how to work out what's right for you? If you're going for the look of a particular era, the charts in this book will show you which colours were in vogue, which go together and which are recommended for your colouring. Most commercial makeup from the twenties to the sixties was aimed at women with ivory to olive skin. If your skin's any darker, that doesn't mean you can't wear vintage looks, just that – in the style of such striking beauties as Josephine Baker (otherwise known as the Black Pearl) – you may have to be a little more creative in adapting them to your own colouring.

WESTMORE'S SEVEN FACE SHAPES

'Most women don't realise that they make a mistake being fashionable, unless the fashion suits their face.'
– *Wally Westmore*

Not all styles suit every face shape: so be prepared to adapt – or even abandon – your favourite looks accordingly. From the 1920s-'60s, the law in this respect was dictated by the Westmores of Hollywood, the dynasty of makeup artists who ruled over almost every studio in town up until the '80s. The five eldest brothers – Monte, Perc, Ern, Wally and Bud – headed up the makeup departments at Selznick, Warner Bros., 20th Century Fox, Paramount and Universal respectively.

Ovalescence was the term coined for perfection of facial form. Agreed upon by experts like Max Factor and the Westmores, this perfect shape was not based on mere visual perceptions but was actually *measurable*. For girls lucky enough to fall into this select group, the aim was to play up their perfectly balanced features. For the rest of womankind, the secret to looking their best was to make their faces appear as oval as possible. In either instance, a careful choice of hairstyle and makeup was vital.

Based around the concept of ovalescence, Perc Westmore built the seven face-shape theory. Every face, he claimed, fit into one of seven

> *'Don't get discouraged if these proportions come out wrong.*
> *Sylvia Sidney's is one face in a thousand where they*
> *come out right. The only thing to do is to give*
> *them the appearance of being balanced.'*
> – Max Factor

categories. By measuring your face at various points you could establish which group you belonged to: triangle, inverted triangle, oblong, round, square, diamond or oval.

For each group, Perc offered a famous poster girl, along with tips on how to emulate her look at home. His theories continued to hold sway and even today you'll find devotees of the seven face-shape theory – or some modern variant – writing beauty columns and styling Hollywood's most gorgeous actresses. So please do take a moment to work out which group you belong to; perhaps by drawing an oval onto a photograph of your face. Can you see which points fall outside the line?

> *'The modern girl achieves*
> *glamour by making the most*
> *of her natural gifts. She*
> *stresses her own good qualities*
> *and minimizes her faults.'*
> – Rita Hayworth

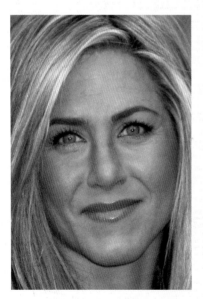

Jennifer Aniston.

1. THE TRIANGLE
Got a strong, broad jaw and a narrow forehead, with your lips as the luscious focal point? This probably makes you a triangle girl.

Your beauty icons: Joan Crawford, Rita Hayworth, Jennifer Aniston

Triangle rules: Sweep hair back from your brow to broaden out your forehead. Avoid short-and-severe crops à la Louise Brooks. Do apply rouge to the highest point of your smile, tapering up towards your temples. Avoid rosebud lip-effects, Cupid's bows . . . anything that would accentuate the wider part of your face.

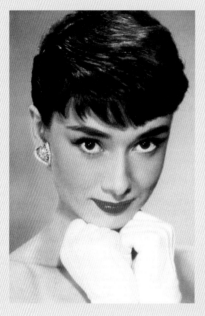

2. THE INVERTED TRIANGLE

If your forehead is broader than your dainty (maybe even pointy) little chin, then why not spotlight your soulful eyes?

Your beauty icons: Audrey Hepburn, Reese Witherspoon, Scarlett Johansson

Inverted triangle rules: Do rouge on the highest point of your cheekbone, sweeping up towards the temples. Create a softly curving lip line to balance out your chin. Keep your eyebrows natural and Hepburn-esque.

Audrey Hepburn.

3. THE OBLONG

In this long, thin shape, you'll find that all outer-points align, with a forehead that's only slightly wider than your chin. The good news for oblong girls is that, as you grow older, your face is destined to hold its shape best of all.

Your beauty icons: Loretta Young, Liv Tyler, Gwyneth Paltrow

Oblong rules: Do wear bangs. They'll shorten your face. Don't arch your brows too steeply – they'll lengthen your face. Don't accentuate the hollows of your cheeks with rouge.

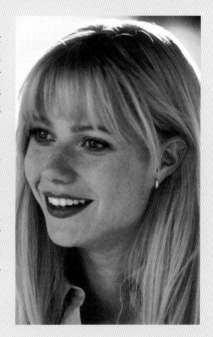

Gwyneth Paltrow.

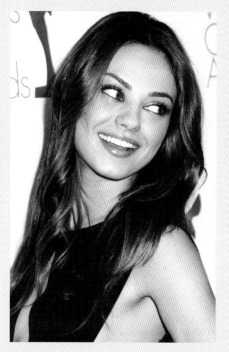

Mila Kunis.

4. THE ROUND FACE

If your hairline and jawline are almost equally broad and your face is at its fullest just below the cheekbones, then your shape is almost certainly round.

Your beauty icons: Lana Turner, Clara Bow, Mila Kunis

Round rules: Don't create straight lines with your hair or makeup. Do pluck your eyebrows in natural arches. Do make up your mouth delicately, emphasising its width. Don't go too light with your foundation; it will make your face look broader. Do apply the darkest rouge you can get away with; sweep across the outer contours of the cheek to add instant shadow.

5. THE DIAMOND

Balancing killer cheekbones with a narrow forehead and chin? Then you're an ever-classy diamond.

Your beauty icons: Katharine Hepburn, Sophia Loren, Olivia Wilde

Diamond rules: Do play down your cheekbones with slightly darker foundation. Do keep eyebrows and lip lines natural, arching in gentle curves. Don't rouge in the hollows of your cheeks.

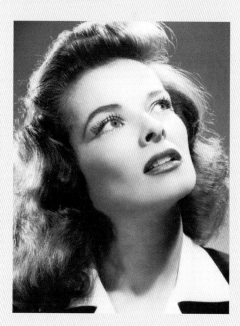

Katharine Hepburn.

6. THE SQUARE

A variation on the oblong, you'll find that all points on the square face align. Jawline and hairline are both square and almost exactly the same width.

Your beauty icons: Grace Kelly, Keira Knightley, Lucy Liu

Square rules: Don't pull hair back too tightly. Wearing it flat on top and/or in tight curls is also best avoided. Do create gentle curves with your brows and lip lines, making your pout as full as possible.

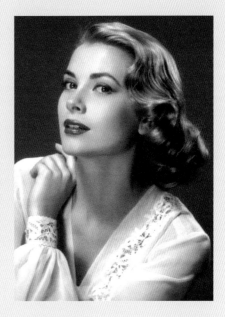

Grace Kelly.

7. THE OVAL

The most desirable of all shapes, oval girls can make the most of their perfectly balanced proportions by avoiding corrective makeup in all its forms.

Your beauty icons: Vivien Leigh, Ava Gardner, Beyoncé

Oval rules: If you're blessed with a widow's peak, brush back your hair and flaunt it. Do create natural-looking, full lips à la Vivien Leigh. Don't overdo it with the rouge. Contouring should not be a part of your beauty regime.

Vivien Leigh.

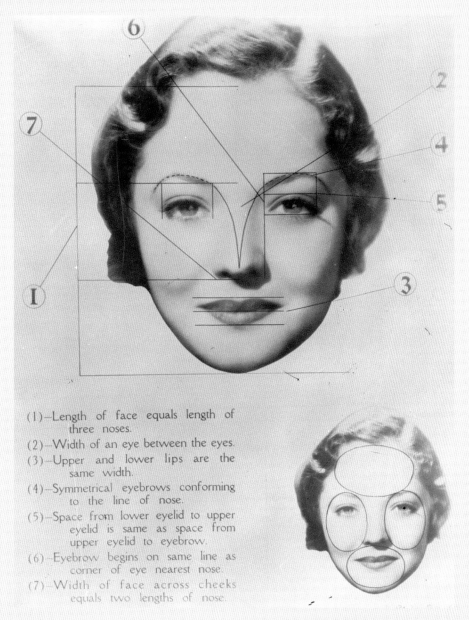

(1)—Length of face equals length of
   three noses.

(2)—Width of an eye between the eyes.

(3)—Upper and lower lips are the
   same width.

(4)—Symmetrical eyebrows conforming
   to the line of nose.

(5)—Space from lower eyelid to upper
   eyelid is same as space from
   upper eyelid to eyebrow.

(6)—Eyebrow begins on same line as
   corner of eye nearest nose.

(7)—Width of face across cheeks
   equals two lengths of nose.

Sylvia Sidney.

A PERFECT OVAL FACE

Although many girls are some variant of this shape – Perc Westmore defined
Bette Davis as a 'round oval', for example – the *perfect* oval face is quite
rare. Film noir stunner Sylvia Sidney and Paulette Goddard (aka Mrs Charlie
Chaplin) are two of a select few girls to meet these exacting standards.

PRACTICE MAKES PERFECT

'What I want you to do is practice putting on your entire makeup . . . Don't expect to blossom out a beauty, as if by magic, just before the doorbell rings at eight Saturday night!'

– Max Factor

Helena Rubinstein would have it that, 'There are no ugly women, only lazy ones'. And there's nothing like practice to help you achieve the look you most desire. In the quest for beauty perfection, Hollywood's leading ladies spent hours in hair and makeup each morning, working with dedicated teams of advisers to create flattering new looks. Experts like Max Factor, the Westmores and Evelyn Marshall of MGM also took the time to teach their charges how to apply their own makeup so that, even out on the street, they continued to represent themselves and the studio in the best possible light.

The best advice these beauty experts had to offer was to examine and experiment. As Joan Crawford put it, stars learnt to study their faces clinically, not emotionally. Don't apply red lipstick because you find the colour seductive but because it suits you. If a colour ages you, throw it away. Work out which shades work for you and how best to apply your mascara to make your eyes seem to open up. Ask yourself, can your lippie hold its own against harsh lighting? According to Max Factor, the eyes and lips are a woman's key features; makeup is all about trying to accentuate them.

'Begin making a fascinating new face for yourself with colours that work into your very own colouring – and see what happens!'

– Joan Crawford

The Westmore brothers were also firm believers in making up *for the occasion.* A candlelit evening and a day at the office clearly require different choices. So, as Mae West would say, 'get the old common sense in action and have a mirror handy'. When you think you've nailed it, Max Factor advises asking the opinion of an honest friend. Did you keep your look natural? Do your best features stand out? Once you've figured out what works for you, it's time to invest in a beauty kit . . .

BUILDING YOUR BEAUTY KIT

'Every woman should know what makeup
she desires and deal with it judicially.'
– Jean Harlow

Whatever your face shape or colouring, there are certain staple products that no girl should be without. Thirties glamour goddess Carole Lombard sums them up:

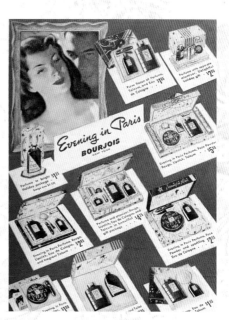

- The three essential creams: night cream, foundation cream, cleansing cream*
- One skin freshener (or ice-cold water)
- Two lipsticks: one for daytime and a brighter shade for evening
- Two rouge compacts: one to serve during the day and a more vivid one for night
- Two boxes of powder: one for day and one for evening. One large puff and one face-powder brush to help you apply them
- Makeup blender for the arms and shoulders
- Eye shadow

- Eyebrow pencil
- Eyelash makeup

*Author's note: If you're unsure what to go for, Pond's cold cream – a Hollywood favourite which first went on sale in the 1840s – will serve in place of all three.

Top tip! Max Factor recommended buying a box with separate compartments for your daytime and evening makeup and for your brushes: 'That way they do not roll around in the drawer and get "snowed under" so that you forget to use them!'

BEAUTY ON THE GO

Whether you're anticipating a long day on-set, or hoping your Friday will take you from water-cooler to dance-floor, there's a secret to makeup that lasts. Here's what Max Factor recommends slipping into your handbag for twenty-four-hour beauty perfection:

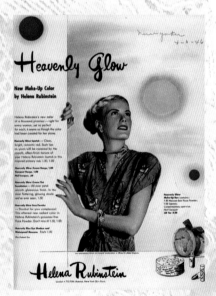

- Eye shadow and powder
- Rouge and lipstick
- Hand cream
- Face cream to remove dirty marks quickly
- A small bottle of eau de Cologne (for a quick pick-me-up)

'A little eau de Cologne will not only ease that tired feeling, but it will wrap you in a subtle fragrance that's most enticing.'
– Max Factor

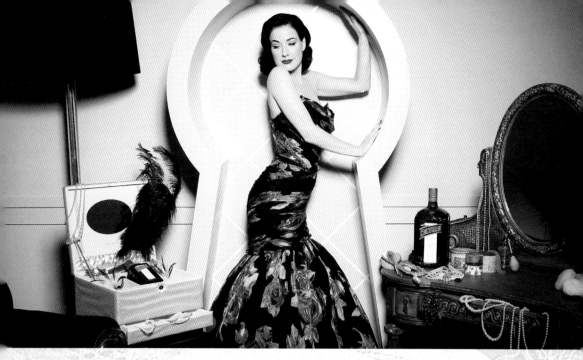

Dita Von Teese.

THE BEAUTY BUDGET

'I advocate glamour. Every day. Every minute.'
– Dita Von Teese

Forget pounds and pence. It's seconds and minutes that count. Flawless thirties sirens like Rochelle Hudson worked out their own personal beauty budgets – allowing time for each and every daily routine – ensuring they'd never be caught unprepared. Here's how you can do the same:

1. Write down every beauty routine you have.
2. Write down how often you need to do them and how long they take.
    For example: Mani-pedi . . . once a week . . . half an hour
    Eye makeup . . . every morning . . . five minutes
    Eye makeup . . . on a night out . . . fifteen minutes
3. Once you've worked out how much time you need to dedicate to glamour, write these routines down on paper, stick them to your mirror or bedside table, and keep to them.

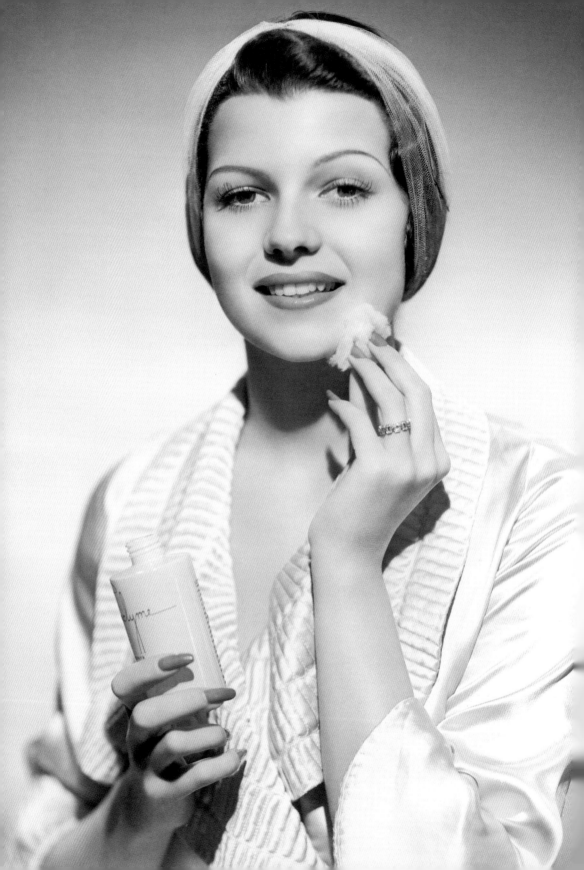

Making Faces

CLEAR COMPLEXIONS

*'There's one thing that stands out above all others
in making a girl really alluring. It's lovely skin.'*
– Clara Bow

Radiant, blemish-free skin is the best canvas for any makeup. Yet achieving this look can be a challenge, even if you happen to be a goddess-like Hollywood siren. Audrey Hepburn confessed to emerging from nearly all her movies as 'a mass of blemishes'. 'I'm fighting problems all the time,' she sighed. After many hours caked in greasepaint, beneath hot studio lighting, it's not surprising that these girls held strong views on how best to battle unsightly breakouts.

Liquefying cleansing creams first came onto the market in the 1920s and remained in vogue until the late thirties. These creams were based on mineral oil and applied with tissues or linen cloths in the same way that Liz Earle's hot-cloth cleanser is used today (this much-loved product is loaded with mineral-only sun filters). The trick was to keep applying the cleanser until you were sure you were really clean because, as Bette Davis warns, 'when you use makeup over a period of years and you don't get it all out, your skin can be ruined'. An astringent lotion was then applied to remove any lingering grease. For added glow (or perhaps because the creams had a tendency to go off in

'I never use water on my face – haven't for about five years. I cleanse it with cold cream, which doesn't dry the skin as water does.'
– Gloria Swanson

Rita Hayworth.

the Californian heat) stars like Fay Wray recommended storing your creams in ice when you weren't using them. Taking it one step further, Jean Harlow rubbed her cream onto ice cubes before applying it to her face; she believed this doubled its effectiveness.

'I have one rule I believe in.
Be sure you get every bit of makeup off at night!'
– Bette Davis

Baby oil was another popular makeup remover – Marlene Dietrich's luminous skin is a wonderful advert for this method. Though you had to be sure to scrub off any greasy residue with soap and water, it seems the oil counteracted the soap's drying effect brilliantly. Hollywood's water was notoriously hard and some stars, like Greta Garbo and Merle Oberon, preferred to wash with softened water. Merle even had a 'water softener' installed in her house. If you don't have a softener of your own, Veronica Lake recommends a squeeze of lemon juice as a natural alternative.

During the war years, when supplies were scarce, soap was the most popular cleanser, applied with a complexion brush to 'stimulate' circulation. Alkaline or bland soaps – especially by Lux – got the Hollywood seal of approval as these were less drying. Most girls, however, borrowed Dad's shaving soap as this was the mildest on the shelves. Many beauty experts swore by this routine for all but the driest of skins, and stars like Marilyn Monroe remained soap-and-water devotees long after cleansers came back into fashion.

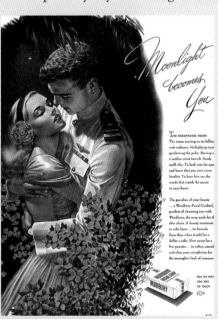

'There's nothing like your face, scrubbed with soap and water.'
– Marilyn Monroe

Available from as early as the mid-nineteenth century, cold cream – whether Woodbury's or Pond's –

RITA HAYWORTH starring in "PAL JOEY"

AN ESSEX-GEORGE SIDNEY PRODUCTION®. A COLUMBIA RELEASE IN TECHNICOLOR®

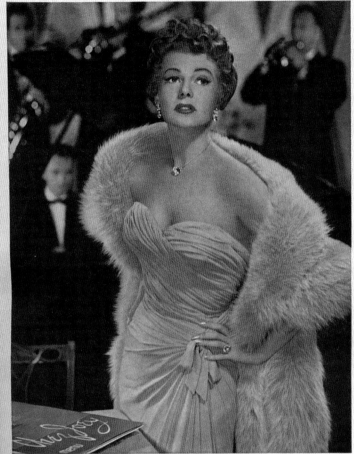

"I always use Lux because it's so gentle, so good to my skin. And I love all four of the new pastel colors" ... *Rita Hayworth*

Now—four more colorful reasons to use Lux!

And pure white Lux sealed in gold foil

Color does something for <u>you</u>
...and so does a lovely complexion!

Lux can do as much for *you* as it does for Rita Hayworth. That's because gentle Lux has a rich *Cosmetic lather*, to help smooth and *soften* your skin.

Soft is the word for the new Lux Colors, too. One or more of these pastels is sure to contrast or harmonize with your bath-room. Use Lux in Color—right along with pure white Lux. (Naturally, you get the same wonderful Lux fragrance!) Lever Brothers guarantees Lux is perfect for your skin—or your money back.

For a complexion you'll love—and he'll love, too—use gentle Lux.

9 out of 1O Hollywood stars depend on LUX

27

also remained a favourite decade after decade (you can still buy it now). Another mineral-oil-based cleanser, cold cream was thicker than liquefying or vanishing creams. You could even leave it on as a night-time moisturiser – at the risk of putting off your hubby. To increase the benefits, Clara Bow liked to give herself a facial massage as she applied her cold cream. Thanks to this regime, she found she could ride in her car with the top down and the wind in her face and still keep a soft, smooth complexion.

Top tip! Hedy Lamarr always went at least one day a week without makeup; she said it gave her skin chance to breathe.

Vintage inspiration: Coconut oil may be one of the hottest beauty trends around today, but back in the thirties, it was Mae West's healthiest obsession. The sexy siren was a vocal advocate of applying it liberally to her face, with obvious benefits. Paul Novak – the love of Mae's life and a former Mr California – was almost thirty years her junior!

Left: *Greta Garbo*. Right: *Ginger Rogers*.

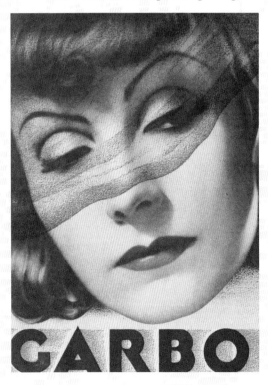

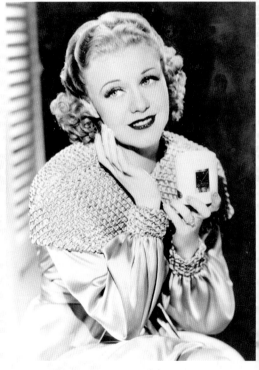

GRETA GARBO'S 'WATER CURE'

'I believe in the water cure. Nothing in the world is better than water, both internally and externally.'
– Greta Garbo

- To give your skin its 'tonic', wash with softened water morning and night. Follow with 'a very light cold cream'.
- Take cold showers to tone your skin.
- Take lukewarm baths to keep your skin soft.
- Apply ice to your face: 'this keeps the muscles from sagging'.
- Drink twelve glasses of water a day for a blemish-free complexion.

HOMEMADE BEAUTY TREATMENTS – CALORIE-FREE INDULGENCES FROM THE KITCHEN CUPBOARD

Wholesome Ginger Rogers based her beauty regime on recipes handed down from her mother. Her favourites included:

- A honey facial: massage with liquid honey, leave on for fifteen to twenty minutes and then rinse off with warm water. According to Ginger, it spells death to blackheads. 'Don't ask me why, because I don't know!'
- Egg-white astringent: smooth the white of an egg over your face; let it dry and harden. This tightens the skin and stimulates circulation. Next, Ginger says, 'just wash it off with cool water – and you'll feel "like a million dollars"'.

If you were wondering what to do with the yolks from the previous recipe, you might try Ava Gardner's trusty preparation below . . .

- Ava's egg-yolk facemask: mix egg yolks with almond oil and apply liberally to the face. Leave this for ten to fifteen minutes to 'work its nourishing magic' then wash off with lukewarm water. Finish with a splash of cold water.

FOUNDATION AND POWDER

'Every makeup requires a background. Something that serves to give a faint colour tone that's uniform to the entire face and to blot out small blemishes.'

– Max Factor

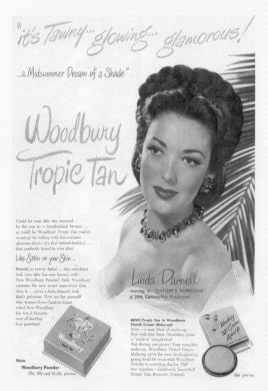

Even if you're going for Ginger's fresh-faced look, that doesn't mean leaving the house without foundation and powder – no glamour girl would. Whether you're a frosty femme who suits cool tones (Marlene Dietrich, Jean Harlow) or a sultry siren (Sophia Loren, Josephine Baker), the one rule insisted upon by experts of all eras is as follows: choose a foundation that matches your natural skin tone. Further adjustments to your colouring can be made at the powder stage. So if you're pale and wishing you could achieve a natural sun-kissed glow, the trick is to apply your foundation first and then add a darker powder over the top (or, even better, a blend of powder and bronzer).

TIPS FOR SILKY-SMOOTH COVERAGE

1. Blend your foundation with fingers dipped in cold water.
2. Always use the bare minimum of foundation. Start by applying to your forehead, cheeks and chin, and blend from there.

3. For flawless coverage, pay extra attention to your hairline, jawline and neck. As Constance Worth says, 'the illusion of powdered daintiness will be completely lost if you don't take care; never, never forget to powder your neck to match your face'.
4. Remember to brush off excess powder. You can use a clean mascara wand or toothbrush to dust off your brows and lashes.
5. If your skin tone changes with the season, so should your makeup.

Top tip! Dolores del Río says: 'Just before you leave the glass, dust your face with a powder a shade darker than the one applied earlier; this will give the skin a "translucent" look.'

Vintage inspiration: Brunette bombshell Jennifer Love Hewitt shared her secret for magical date nights. 'Elizabeth Taylor taught me that if you do your hair and makeup first then take a hot bath right before you leave, it brings out your inner glow and takes away the powdery look from makeup. I do that right before every date.'

APPLYING 'WARMTH' (ROUGE)

'Know your complexion. There's a rouge to match it that's as skilfully blended by scientists as the pigments are by famous painters. Don't spoil the effect then, by being satisfied with an "off-tone". You wouldn't like it on canvas. Why do it to yourself?'
– Max Factor

Today's blusher comes in many luxurious forms, whether liquid, cream or powder. While you may wish to stay true to the twenties and load up your powder puff, it's possible to create more subtle effects – that don't rub off so easily – with a cream or liquid rouge (advisable if you're going for dewy radiance rather than matte perfection).

TIPS FOR RAVISHING ROUGE

1. Select your perfect match. From bold scarlet to a touch of rose, raspberry shimmer to rich geranium, you're sure to find a shade that complements your colouring. Refer back to Helena Rubinstein's colour charts and prepare to reap the benefits.
2. Apply lightly to begin with; you can always add more.
3. When applying powdered rouge, always start at the temples and work down.
4. For cream or liquid rouge, apply in upward circular motions and use a light touch.
5. Blend well to avoid a visible line, especially with cream rouge.
6. Powder over your rouge for more subtle colour.

CONTOURING WITH ROUGE

A girl's best friend, rouge can be used to correct or disguise a multitude of features.

Wishing for a fuller-looking face? Adding rouge to the apples of your cheeks (the parts that rise up when you smile) should have the desired effect. Just be sure to steer clear of your nose. According to Jack Dawn – head of makeup at MGM – applying colour in a horizontal motion also helps add width to thinner faces.

Want to downplay your 'moon' face? Rouging close to your nose will spotlight the centre of your face, giving you the illusion of length. Apple-cheeked Clara Bow never failed to follow this rule.

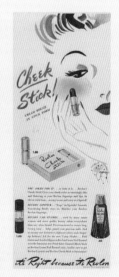

To fill out your cheeks, avoid rouging in the hollow where the colour will act as a shadow, accentuating the drawn-in look. Instead, start at the cheekbones and blend round the outline of the face, making it appear fuller.

Feeling less than fabulous? For an instant pick-me-up, try bringing your rouge a little higher than usual, adding a light dusting under your eyes. According to Max Factor, 'this not only gives the eyes an extra sparkle, but it does away with those white spaces or dark rings, as the case may be, immediately below them'.

Top tip! To play up her elegant cheekbones, Grace Kelly used two different shades of rouge – a light luminous tone over the bone and a darker dusting in the hollows below. This simple but stunning trick has been imitated by everyone from Kim Kardashian to Emma Watson. 'I like a blush because I am so pale and English,' the beauty once quipped.

DRAMATIC EFFECTS:
LIGHTS AND SHADOWS

'As a child, perhaps you were amused by optical illusions . . . as an adult seeking loveliness, the theories they demonstrate can help you to work makeup magic in your face.'
– Westmore Beauty Book

Contouring – using makeup to spotlight certain features while causing others to recede – is a time-honoured Hollywood trick that's particularly effective in black and white. As the *Westmore Beauty Book* explains: 'light reflects light' while 'shadow absorbs' it. Ergo, it pays to add a little radiance to the finer points of your bone structure (with product like MAC's wondrous Strobe Cream), while downplaying other areas with darker-toned foundation. Thanks to the

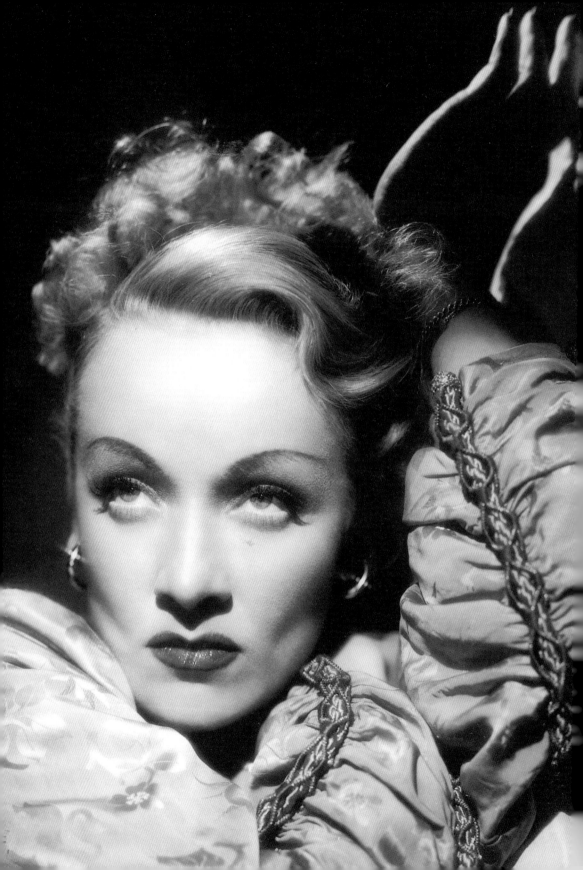

range of darker bases (for adding shadow) and shimmery highlighters available today (in a range of tones from ethereal white through to lustrous gold) it's easy for the average girl to make the most of her bone structure. Here's how you can create dramatic shadows and brilliant highlights of your own . . .

- By highlighting her fabulous, feline cheekbones, Sophia Loren was able to draw the eye away from her long nose. You can achieve her sculpted look by sweeping highlighter across your cheekbones and up towards your temples. For added Mediterranean glow, opt for a product that has warm golden undertones.
- Marlene Dietrich drew a fine white or silver line down the centre of her nose to make it appear straighter. She used white greasepaint along the inside line of her lower lashes to make her eyes appear wider (white eyeliner would work just as well). She also applied rouge within the hollows of her cheeks to accentuate her already drawn-in look. Of course, determined Dietrich is rumoured to have had her molar teeth removed in an effort to emphasise her amazingly sculpted cheekbones. Thanks to the invention of satiny pink highlighter creams like Girl Meets Pearl by Benefit (which you can sweep across your cheekbones to gorgeous effect), there's no reason for modern girls to go to surgical extremes.
- Claudette Colbert used a darker shade of foundation on her prominent cheekbones.
- *La Dolce Vita* siren Anita Ekberg used dark shadowing to soften her angular jawline.

Modern-day master class: Reality TV star Kim Kardashian is the queen of contouring and has never been shy about sharing her expertise with the world. 'How do I look?' she tweeted one day, posting a picture of her face with bright white highlighter drawn neatly down her nose, fanning out across her forehead and outlining her trademark sculpted cheekbones. Several hours and layers of bronzer later, and KK was red-carpet-ready for the cameras.

Marlene Dietrich.

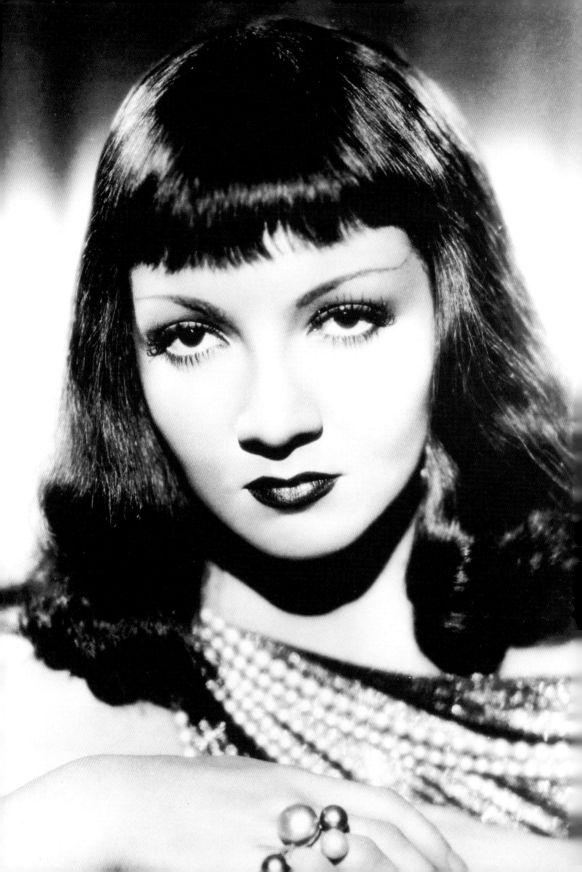

Lip Tips

'Get as close as possible to the nearest
mirror and look at your mouth, lady!'
– Dorothy Lamour

VINTAGE COLOURS AND STYLES

1920s: dark red lips, drawn in a delicate rosebud or tiny bee-stung shape, predominated in the era of Mae Murray and Clara Bow.
Modern-day master class: Lily Cole. Lily's china-white complexion contrasts beautifully with her dainty crimson pout.

1930s: girls of this decade were natural, favouring rose pinks and soft reds by day, and 'tropical' orange-based reds and coral pinks in the evening. Bracket lips (with curves on the top and bottom) à la Jean Harlow gave way to hunter's bows (aka 'the Joan Crawford smear').
Modern-day master class: Emma Stone. Revlon's poster girl of the moment is often seen rocking vibrant coral lips, proving that red is not the only colour for full-on evening glam.

1940s: in the 1940s, lips could be any shade you liked – so long as that shade was red! This trend was mostly inspired

THE PERFECT KISS
PAMPERING BALM WITH
LIGHTWEIGHT STAIN

NEW REVLON JUST BITTEN KISSABLE™ BALM STAIN

Get smoother, softer looking lips with a perfect flush of color that will last hour after hour, in all 12 vibrant shades. No Sharpener required.

REVLON

Revlon.com

Claudette Colbert.

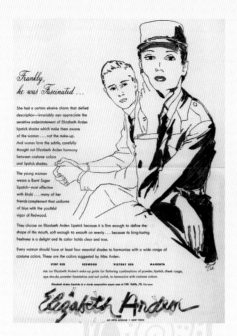

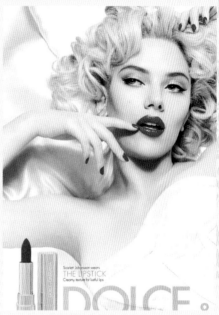

by Elizabeth Arden who designed a series of
lipsticks for servicewomen, in shades to match
the fiery chevrons on their uniforms. Pin-up
girls like Rita Hayworth and Betty Grable
showed off the look to its best advantage.

Modern-day master class: Scarlett
Johansson. Scarlett's enviable pillow lips are
rarely seen without a swipe of her favourite
shade by Dolce & Gabbana. 'Their Classic
Cream Lipstick in Devil is perfect,' says
Scarlett. 'Not too blue and not too orange . .
. it always makes me feel good.'

1950s: bright corals and pinks were the
vogue. Lips were drawn into a larger version
of the twenties rosebud shape with plenty
of curve.

Modern-day master class: Christina
Hendricks. Christina's vibrant coral lips
– regularly painted with Julie Hewett's
luxurious Bijou Collection Lipstick in Celeste
– are stolen straight from her character in *Mad
Men*, proving we can all learn a thing or two
from kittenish office angel Joan Holloway.

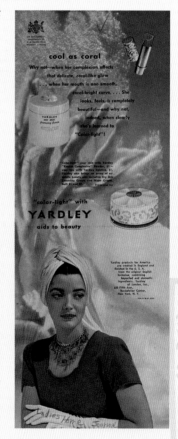

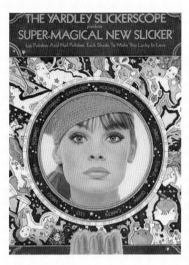

THE YARDLEY SLICKERSCOPE
predicts
SUPER-MAGICAL NEW SLICKER
Lip Polishes And Nail Polishes. Each Shade To Make You Lucky In Love

1960s: sixties makeup was all about the eyes, played up by pairs of very pale lips. Pastels in all colours were popular (yes, even green) with an almost whited-out look favoured at the beginning of the decade. Brown and beige were the colours of choice for summer. This decade also saw the arrival of the very first lip-glosses. The exciting new trend for 'slicker' (as worn on-screen by beautiful Italian film stars) allowed girls to add shine without colour for the first time ever.

Modern-day master class: Lana Del Rey. The chanteuse's glossy nude lips and Bambi eyes are the epitome of sixties style. Lana's barely-there lipstick of choice – Blond Ingénu by YSL – provides the perfect contrast to her striking winged eyeliner.

PAINTING PERFECT LIPS

Favoured by Elizabeth Taylor *and* Joan Crawford, this is the only method you need to know!

You will need:
- Lip brush (or orangewood stick)
- Lip rouge (the kind that is applicable with a brush)
- Lipstick – with enough pigment to hide the natural contours of your lips
- A dusting of your favourite finishing powder
1. Start with smooth, exfoliated lips; this ensures more even coverage.
2. Trace around your lips with a small brush loaded with your colour of choice, using firm clear outlines to create the shape that you desire.
3. Fill in the outline with your lipstick, blending with your fingers. Be sure to rub well towards the inside of the mouth to avoid a noticeable line.

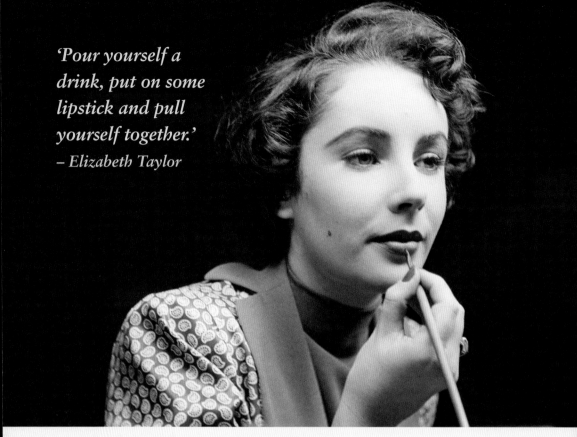

'Pour yourself a drink, put on some lipstick and pull yourself together.'
– Elizabeth Taylor

Elizabeth Taylor.

4. Press your lips together; blot well with a folded tissue.
5. Dust with finishing powder and apply a second coat of lipstick.
6. Blot again. And you're ready to go!

Top tip! Don't skip the blotting stage. It's far better for the excess to come off on the tissue and not your cup or cigarette. According to *Hollywood* beauty editor Mary Bailey, those tell-tale red rings were one of the biggest pet peeves amongst servicemen.

CONTOURING FOR KISSABLE LIPS

'Even when I'm at home alone,
I wear my lipstick. I feel naked without it.'
– Bette Davis

To fill out thinner lips, pencil over the natural lip line and fill your voluptuous new shape with matching lipstick. Gorgeous Vivien Leigh spent her working life plumping out her lower lip in this manner. Her petulant performance in *Gone with the Wind* – as Southern-belle-from-hell, Scarlett O'Hara – is testament to the wondrous impact of just a little extra liner. Your perfect pout: Vivien Leigh.

- To make a large mouth appear smaller, don't paint quite to the edges of your lips. Try using a deeper colour in the centre of your lips and lightening outwards. Your perfect pout: Joan Blondell.
- To make full lips appear thinner, keep the colour well within the natural lip line and use 'contrast lighting'. The upper lip should be a shade darker than the lower one. Your perfect pout: Sophia Loren.
- Drooping lips: 'Don't make up the corners. Stop the colour at the point where they start to droop,' says Ginger Rogers. Your perfect pout: Ginger Rogers.

Modern-day master class: To create the most luscious pout in history, Marilyn Monroe is rumoured to have layered her lips with up to five different shades of colour. Using darker hues at the edges, Marilyn saved the most vibrant, traffic-stopping reds for the centre, making her a source of lip-inspiration for generations to come. Karin Darnell – makeup artist to sultry songstress Rihanna – recently revealed that 'for the "Ti Amo" video I used a deep, dark berry lipstick with a gloss in the middle of the lip to break it up. Light in the centre, whether it's a clear gloss or a hint of pink or red, will give dark lip colours warmth' – a perfect tip for those wishing to rock a less severe version of the vampy, Bordeaux-stained shades of the twenties.

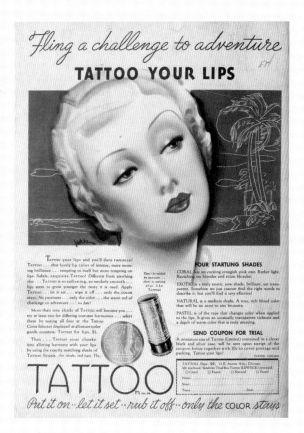

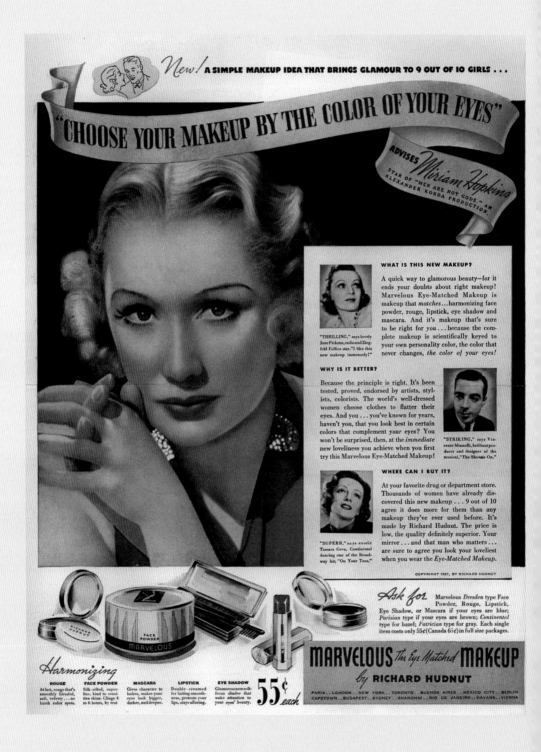

New! A SIMPLE MAKEUP IDEA THAT BRINGS GLAMOUR TO 9 OUT OF 10 GIRLS . . .

"CHOOSE YOUR MAKEUP BY THE COLOR OF YOUR EYES"

ADVISES *Miriam Hopkins*
STAR OF "MEN ARE NOT GODS," AN ALEXANDER KORDA PRODUCTION

"THRILLING," says lovely Jane Pickens, radiant and Ziegfeld Follies star. "I like this new makeup immensely!"

"SUPERB," says exotic Tamara Geva, Continental dancing star of the Broadway hit, "On Your Toes."

WHAT IS THIS NEW MAKEUP?

A quick way to glamorous beauty—for it ends your doubts about right makeup! Marvelous Eye-Matched Makeup is makeup that *matches*...harmonizing face powder, rouge, lipstick, eye shadow and mascara. And it's makeup that's sure to be right for *you*...because the complete makeup is scientifically keyed to your own personality color, the color that never changes, *the color of your eyes!*

WHY IS IT BETTER?

Because the principle is right. It's been tested, proved, endorsed by artists, stylists, colorists. The world's well-dressed women choose clothes to flatter their eyes. And you ... you've known for years, haven't you, that you look best in certain colors that complement *your eyes?* You won't be surprised, then, at the *immediate* new loveliness you achieve when you first try this Marvelous Eye-Matched Makeup!

"STRIKING," says Vincente Minnelli, brilliant producer and designer of the musical, "The Show is On."

WHERE CAN I BUY IT?

At your favorite drug or department store. Thousands of women have already discovered this new makeup . . . 9 out of 10 agree it does more for them than any makeup they've ever used before. It's made by Richard Hudnut. The price is low, the quality definitely superior. Your mirror . . . and that man who matters . . . are sure to agree you look your loveliest when you wear the *Eye-Matched Makeup.*

COPYRIGHT 1937, BY RICHARD HUDNUT

Ask for Marvelous *Dresden* type Face Powder, Rouge, Lipstick, Eye Shadow, or Mascara if your eyes are blue; *Parisian* type if your eyes are brown; *Continental* type for hazel; *Patrician* type for gray. Each single item costs only 55¢ (Canada 65¢) in full size packages.

Harmonizing

ROUGE	FACE POWDER	MASCARA	LIPSTICK	EYE SHADOW
At last, rouge that's smoothly blended, soft, velvety . . . no harsh color spots.	Silk-sifted, superfine, kind to sensitive skins. Clings 4 to 6 hours, by test.	Gives character to lashes, makes your eyes look bigger, darker, and deeper.	Double-creamed for lasting smoothness, protects your lips, stays alluring.	Glamorous new soft-focus shades that wake attention to your eyes' beauty.

55¢ *each*

MARVELOUS *The Eye-Matched* MAKEUP
by RICHARD HUDNUT

PARIS . LONDON . NEW YORK . TORONTO . BUENOS AIRES . MEXICO CITY . BERLIN
CAPETOWN . BUDAPEST . SYDNEY . SHANGHAI . RIO DE JANEIRO . HAVANA . VIENNA

FACE POWDER MARVELOUS

42

The Eyes
Have It

*'Even naturally beautiful eyes are
improved by the right makeup.'*
– *Alberto de Rossi*

Audrey Hepburn once described a woman's eyes as 'the doorway to her heart' – as the sirens of vintage Hollywood understood better than anyone. From smouldering twenties sirens who never had to speak to say 'come hither' to doe-eyed sixties ingénues, read on for details of how to showcase your most enchanting facial feature vintage-style . . .

CHOOSING YOUR
COLOUR AND STYLE

1920s: sultry, smoky shades and lashings of kohl.
1930s: classy neutral hues (beige and champagne) for daywear; shimmery metallic shades for added evening glamour.
1940s: blue, grey, blue-grey, brown, green and violet. Mix blue and violet to get a shade of lilac to match your fashionable hat!
1950s: strong colours – blues, greens, pinks and violets.
1960s: pretty pastels, topped with heavy eyeliner and mascara.

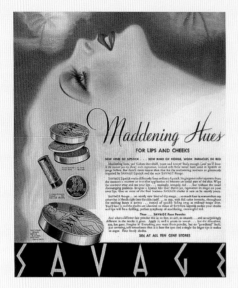

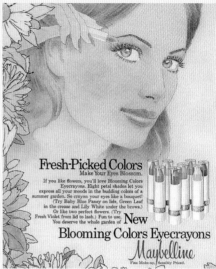

Top tip! Rest those peepers. To keep her big, blue eyes twinkling, Bette Davis rested cucumber slices on her lids every night before bed. She also wore petroleum jelly under her eyes to protect against puffiness and dark circles overnight. Other actresses used cotton pads drenched in soothing lotion, à la Janet Leigh.

MASCARA

'Every woman needs a man who will ruin
her lipstick and not her mascara.'
– Marilyn Monroe

APPLICATION TIPS

1. Always apply to the upper lashes first, using an upward stroke to add curl.
2. Go lightly with your lower lashes – using too much can create shadow under your eyes. Fabulous Fraulein Marlene Dietrich never wore any mascara at all on her lower lashes for this very reason.

3. For added evening drama, let the mascara dry and then apply a second layer – you'll need it under those artificial lights.

4. Take time to separate your lashes when you're done, using an eyelash comb or – in the style of wide-eyed beauty Audrey Hepburn – a single pin.

HOW TO USE CAKE MASCARA

Once upon a time, mascara came in the form of a solid block rather than a handbag-friendly tube. For those girls committed to an authentically vintage look – with not a clump in sight – *The Polly Bergen Book of Beauty, Fashion and Charm* explains how to apply cake mascara like a pro.

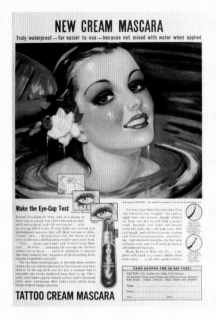

You will need:
- Cake mascara
- A mascara brush
- A second mascara brush which you will have cut jagged with nail scissors so that some of the bristles are long and some short

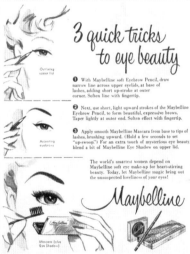

1. Wet the brush. Then take off excess water with a tissue until the brush is almost dry.
2. Rub the brush over the cake mascara, then use the tissue to remove any excess so that you are beginning with *an almost dry brush*.
3. Flick your lashes upwards. Then, while that eye is drying, do the same with the other eye. Keep going over the lashes until you get the look you want.
4. Take the jagged brush (dry) and use it to separate the lashes.

EYELASH RULES:
1. Daytime mascara should be black for brunettes and brown for blondes and redheads.
2. Don't overdo it. As Marilyn Monroe points out, 'when a man looks into your eyes, he doesn't like looking into a mess of mascara!' If ever you over-apply, use a dry brush to take off the excess.
3. There's no shame in faking it – Bette Davis always wore false lashes and her eyes were striking enough to have inspired their own song.
4. Never apply fake lashes too near to the nose. According to Italo Fava, head of Max Factor's Parisian salon in the 1960s, this will make your eyes look closer together.
5. Never apply false lashes straight from the box; they should always be trimmed to fit, advised Elizabeth Arden's Creative Director, Pablo Manzoni in 1960.

Top tip! Lucille Ball recommends applying castor oil to the lashes at night to help keep them thick and glossy. Face cream was another popular lash treatment.

EYELINER

Seeking a way to highlight, define and instantly open up your eyes to the world? Then – like generations of vintage vixens before you – you're in need of a classic black liner. Of course, the sirens of the silver screen have flirted with various styles throughout Hollywood history. To recreate the sultry look of the twenties, you'll need to go heavy on the kohl, yet the forties girl wore almost none. The thirties fashion for outlining both the eye and the eye socket is mirrored by the fashions of the sixties. Flirty fifties girls usually went for a single line along the upper lash. Whichever look you choose to channel, it pays to remember the basics:

1. Lining all around your eyes will make them appear smaller.
2. A line along the top of your eye socket will make your eyes look deeper-set.
3. Never, ever wear eyeliner without mascara; it will make the line too obvious.

4. Blend sultry shades of eyeliner up over the lid for a dramatic, smoky look.

Top tip! To create her famous smoky eyes, Marlene Dietrich held a lighted match under a saucer, then mixed the resulting soot with baby oil and applied to her lids. The trick was to start with a dark line near the roots of the lashes and blend upwards to almost nothing at the top of the lid. If you don't fancy her dicey, fire-starting method, you could always substitute Marlene's soot for liquid liner or dark (almost midnight black) eye shadow mixed with baby oil.

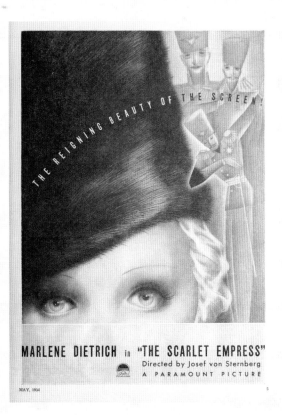

MARLENE DIETRICH in "THE SCARLET EMPRESS"
Directed by Josef von Sternberg
A PARAMOUNT PICTURE

EYE SHADOW

'Your eye shadow will do wonders if you'll let it.'
– Max Factor

GENERAL RULES:
- Apply with a brush and use your fingers to blend, blend, blend.
- For a daytime look, Max Factor advises you use only as much eye shadow as you need to complement your gorgeous natural colouring. 'For instance, Claudette Colbert can use a great deal of brown eye shadow with her brown eyes without making it obvious,

while a light application of grey is all Ann Harding needs to make her blue eyes infinitely more blue.'

- In the evenings, there are no rules! From Josephine Baker's smoky black sockets and Brigitte Bardot's bold winged shape, to Greta Garbo's flawlessly contoured come-to-bed eyes, there's no limit as to the effects you can create with combinations of your favourite shades.

Top tip! Dorothy Lamour always topped her bright eye shadow with a coat of foundation, to give only 'the faintest glimmering of colour . . . subtle but effective.'

EYEBROWS

'The perfect eyebrow starts at the point above the inner corner of the eye. Its arch should follow the curve of the eye socket.'
– Bette Davis

Eyebrow fashions changed dramatically from the twenties to the sixties, getting broader and bushier as the decades went on. Whether you choose to frame your eyes with the pencil-thin arch of a twenties flapper, the straight and severe lines of the thirties, the more natural forties look or the bushy-and-beautiful shapes of the sixties is up to you – just so long as you remember these vintage guidelines:

Finding your ideal brow length. Flick back to Perc Westmore's diagram of the ideal oval face and you'll see your brow should start in line with your tear duct. Can you trace a line from your nose, across the corner of your eye to the tip of your brow? If your brows are too short, extend them with pencil. If they're too long, pluck 'em.

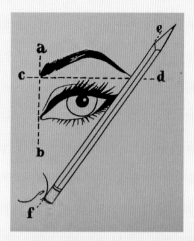

And your perfect pitch. When shaping your brows, divide the length of your eyebrow into imaginary quarters, advises Polly Bergen. Your 'high point' should be at the three-quarter mark – usually lining up with the outer edge of the iris.

EYEBROW RULES:
- Never pluck against the grain!
- Never tweeze above the brow. Brush the hairs upward and then pluck from below, following the natural curve of your eye.
- Never touch the inner-corner of your brow, says Paramount's 'Mr Makeup' Eddie Senz; the lower it dips, the higher your arch will look.
- Don't over-pluck, advises Alberto de Rossi, the makeup artist responsible for shaping Audrey Hepburn's famously beautiful brows.
- When selecting an eyebrow pencil, never go more than a shade lighter or darker than your natural brows. If you're a blonde, take Mae West as your example; her come-hither glances wouldn't have been half so seductive from under thick black brows!

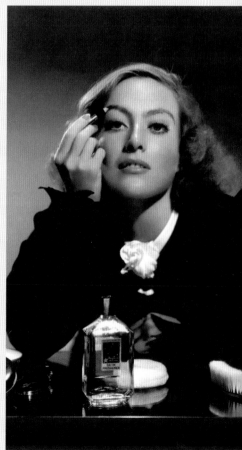

Joan Crawford.

- Rather than 'colouring in' your brows, build them up using soft, diagonal strokes that mimic the hair around them. For an authentically vintage look, try swapping your usual pencil for an angled brush and colour. Maybelline's Ultra Brow Brush-On Color and Illamasqua's Eyebrow Cake are two fantastic products still on the shelves today that can help you shine like a starlet.
- Tidy up. Even natural brows should be neat – straggling hairs are *never* permissible! And for true vintage beauty, why not give them a nightly brush with a little castor oil?

Vintage inspiration: Cara Delevingne and her statement eyebrows have been ruling runways since 2010. But she's far from the first fashion queen to rock bold, beautiful brows. Check out the shape of Audrey Hepburn's brows back in 1954's *Sabrina* and it's easy to see where Cara drew her blocky black inspiration. In both cases, the contrast between the strong black brow and the delicate features beneath is truly striking.

Cara Delevingne.

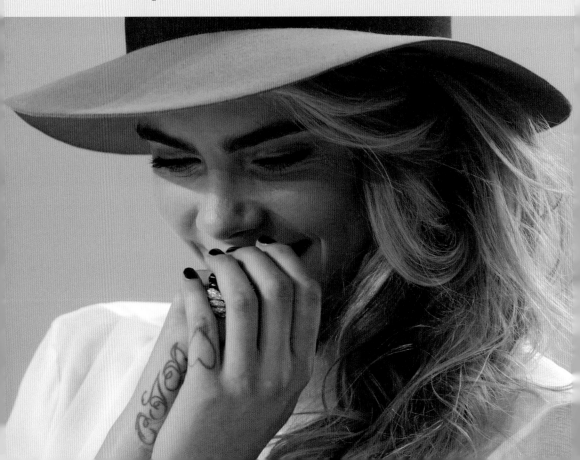

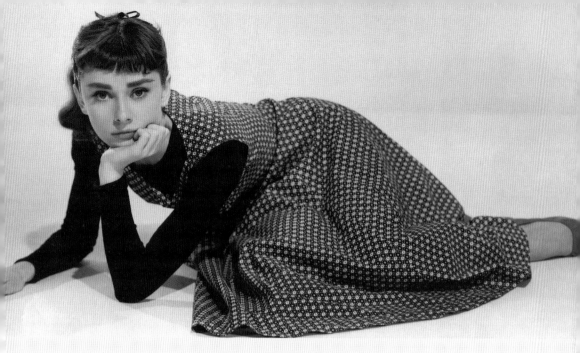

Audrey Hepburn.

WHAT YOUR EYEBROWS SAY ABOUT YOU, BY MAX FACTOR

'Eyebrows are key to the whole facial expression.'
– Max Factor

'**Sophistication,** for instance, is emphasised by a winged eyebrow that sweeps up at the end.

The semi-circle variety – which makes a girl seem eternally surprised – belongs to the **ingénue.** But be careful, for it's apt to cause the eyes to appear quite small.

Straight brows denote **strength** and **efficiency** – although they're deadly on a square-ish face which needs to have them arched.

The most **romantic** kind are the rounded brows which follow the natural bone structure.

Joan Blondell is a **joyous, bubbling** person. Of course, her eyebrows would be slender and delicately arched.'

CORRECTIONAL EYE MAKEUP

	EYEBROWS	MASCARA
SMALL EYES	'Create the illusion of size by arching the eyebrow just a bit lower than usual – but not so low that your expression will be too severe. Remove just a few hairs from the upper edge of the brows; accent the lower arch with the eyebrow pencil.' – Gloria Mack 'The trick is to highlight them from below. So, with tiny even strokes, draw your eyebrow pencil under the lashes of the lower lid – and don't forget to use your fingertip to blend it!' – Max Factor	'Apply a good layer of mascara and then separate out the lashes. Once the mascara has dried, use an eyelash curler to open up the eyes.' – Eddie Senz, Paramount's Mr Makeup
ROUND EYES	'Shape the eyebrow ovally so that there is no feeling of a rounded arch. Always be sure the eyebrow is not thinned too much. Work with the pencil until the eye takes on a definite almond shape.' – Gloria Mack 'With your eyebrow pencil extend the line of the eyebrow a trifle and be careful to make it darker near the nose.' – Max Factor	'Use mascara only on the lashes in the centre of the eyes to the outer corners.' – Gloria Mack 'And put more of the eyelash makeup on your outer lashes.' – Max Factor
LARGE/ PROMINENT EYES	'Don't wear too thin brows; but don't make them too heavy. Make up the lower section of the face so that attention will be immediately drawn to some feature of it.' – Gloria Mack	'Mascara only the upper lashes . . . and very lightly.' – Gloria Mack
DEEP-SET EYES		'Always use plenty of mascara and fake lashes.' – Pablo Manzoni, Elizabeth Arden's Creative Director

'If you will experiment a little, you will discover that a bit of shadow placed at the end of the lid makes your eyes look larger.'

– Ginger Rogers

EYE SHADOW	EYELINER
'Use little eye shadow – and none at all in the hollow of the eyelid next to the nose.' – Gloria Mack Using a little white eye shadow or highlight above and below the eyebrow will make the eyes appear wider.	'Never use eyeliner to line the lids,' says Eddie Senz. However a small amount applied to the very corners of the eyes gives an enlarged look. And certainly, use eye-brightener (or 'eye-lighter' as this white highlighter is sometimes known in the US): 'The trick is to highlight them from below. So with tiny even strokes, draw your eyebrow pencil under the lashes of the lower lid – and don't forget to use your fingertip to blend it!' – Max Factor
'Follow general eye shadow rules: never apply shadow with the same density over the whole lid; never apply it under the eye.' – Gloria Mack	'Extend the line of the upper and lower lids at the outer corner with an eyebrow pencil. Then, with the cushions of your fingertips, blur the line into a scarcely perceptible shadow. That way you get the most natural effects.' – Max Factor
'Blend the eye shadow carefully over the prominent part of the upper lid; use as dark a shade as possible.' – Gloria Mack	'An eyebrow pencil drawn lightly just above the lashes of the upper lid' is all the highlighting large eyes need, according to Max Factor.
'Use light eye shadow.' – Santiago 'Sergio' Seijo, personal makeup artist to Sophia Loren 'Use eye shadow from the centre outward – you get the proper balance of light and shade.' – Max Factor	

PROTECT YOUR NAILS
make them more beautiful
with DURA-GLOSS

Naturally, when your nails are radiant with the sparkling color and gleaming highlights that only Dura-[Gloss] can give them, you'll feel elated, jubilant, *good*! You'll [have] the feeling *of poise, of importance*, that goes with we[aring] Dura-Gloss.

Thousands of women have already switched to Dura-G[loss] and many of them write us that they are amazed at th[e way] Dura-Gloss "*stays with*" their nails for days on end. [Why] not try it yourself today?

Why DURA-GLOSS excels

To produce a polish that yields exceptional wear[,] that does not *chip off* readily, that *dries* har[d] with unparalleled brilliance, the Dura-Glos[s] formula contains a specially formulated resi[n] almost identical to the world's most treasure[d] resins which come from fossilized trees burie[d] deep in the earth since prehistoric times. (Am[-] ber, from which precious jewelry is made is on[e] of these resins . . . cherished for its exceptiona[l] gem-like *hardness* and incomparable *luster*[.] *This is why* Dura-Gloss puts a finish on you[r] nails of such surpassing *brilliance, luster* an[d] *adhesion*. See for yourself what a marvelou[s] polish Dura-Gloss is . . . do it today[!]

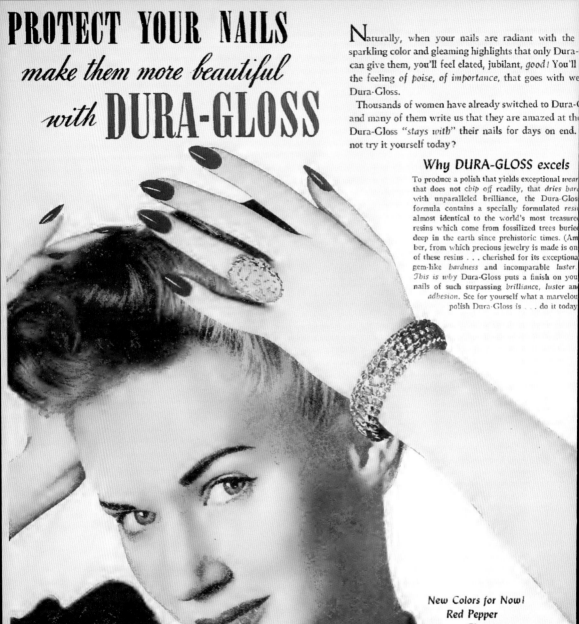

New Colors for Now!
Red Pepper
Cinnamon
Nutmeg

10 PLUS

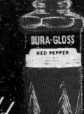

DURA-GLOSS
RED PEPPER

It's DURA-GLOSS *for*
the most beautiful fingernails in the world

Winning Hands

'Your hands . . . what are they saying about you as they move over the coffee pot? Are they white and smooth and cared for? Or dull, hardened "housewife" hands?'
– Max Factor

My beautifully-groomed grandmother taught me that a girl should always pay attention to her hands. On display at all times, they're a huge part of anyone's first impression of you. As much as your face or your hair, your hands send a message to others about who you are and your attention to detail. Here's how to ensure they do you credit . . .

CHOOSING NAIL COLOUR AND STYLE – THE VINTAGE WAY

'It is always a problem what colour nail polish to choose, especially for red-headed girls like me. Red hair and off-shade red nails can fight furiously.'
– Ginger Rogers

1930s: chic by day and exotic by night, the thirties girl-next-door has a split personality. With the invention of metallic polishes and ornaments, nails became longer and ever-more dramatic.

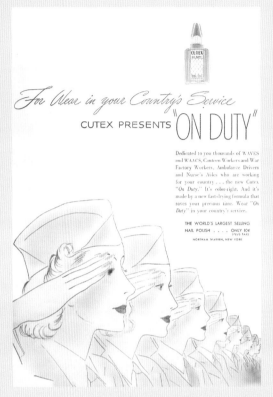

'Presto, change-o! From coral to rust and then to vermilion and wine reds is the morning-to-dusk colour scheme for fingernails of the cinema stars who cleverly tint their nails to complement their costumes.'
– Hollywood *magazine*

1940s: the working girls of the forties filed their nails shorter to match the contour of their fingers. From nine to five, nails were neutral, with more glamorous shades for evenings out.
1950s: nails were longer, darker and most definitely matched your lipstick.
1960s: nude shades and pale pastels were the vogue.

'Shorter fingernails are just more attractive and appealing and will prove far more practical.'
– *Wally Westmore*

MERLE OBERON'S GOLDEN RULES OF NAIL HARMONY

*'I am unconsciously conscious of my hands.
I do give them very good care, but I don't coddle them.
I like to use my hands – do things with them.'*
– *Merle Oberon*

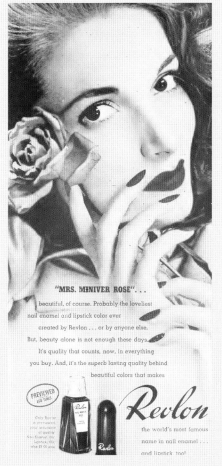

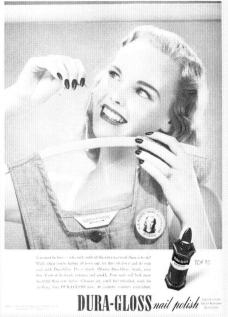

• Paint your nails to match your mood. Indian-born beauty Merle was much sought-after for 'exotic' roles, calling for vampy shades and long, pointed tips. To play a 'more conservative, natural type of girl,' she kept them filed in neat ovals, 'of medium length' with 'untinted' tips.

• Coordinate with your ensemble. Merle's daytime neutrals blend with 'almost any frock'. In the evening – when Merle favoured monochrome gowns – her nails are brighter and more dramatic. In summer, she opts for russet shades to complement her glowing tan.

• Avoid nail-lip clashes at all costs. Thankfully in 1945, Revlon introduced the first range of matching nail and lip colours. Legend has it that the company's founding father, Charles Revlon, came up with the concept whilst dining in a smart restaurant. Appalled, he watched as a finely-dressed woman dabbed her lips with clashing nails. The rest is history.

STELLAR HAND-CARE TIPS
FROM IRENE DUNNE

*'All modern girls appreciate the importance of soft,
smooth hands tipped by glistening nails.'*
– Ann Vernon, Hollywood *magazine*

Another girl with famously beautiful hands was the actress, Irene Dunne. Here's how she kept them silken and supple:

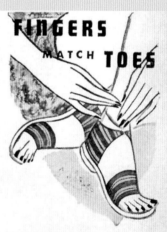

- Don't scrimp on the lotion. Created circa 1930, Elizabeth Arden's Eight Hour Cream is an ever-classy solution to the age-old problem of dry, chapped hands. Apply morning and night, and after drying washes.
- Natural, not neglected! Even unpainted nails should be neatly filed and buffed. Irene recommends letting your hand shape guide you as you file your nails.
- Wear gloves (or else skip the washing up).
- Treat yourself to a weekly manicure.

Irene's piano-scale exercise: lay your hand on a flat surface. Keeping your palm flat on the table, lift each finger in turn, raising it as high as possible and bringing it down with a tap. Repeat with the other hand.

Interlaced piano scales: place one hand on top of the other with interlacing fingers. Stretch them as far and as wide as you can. Then, follow the piano-scale exercise as above, always keeping your fingers interlaced.

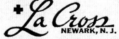

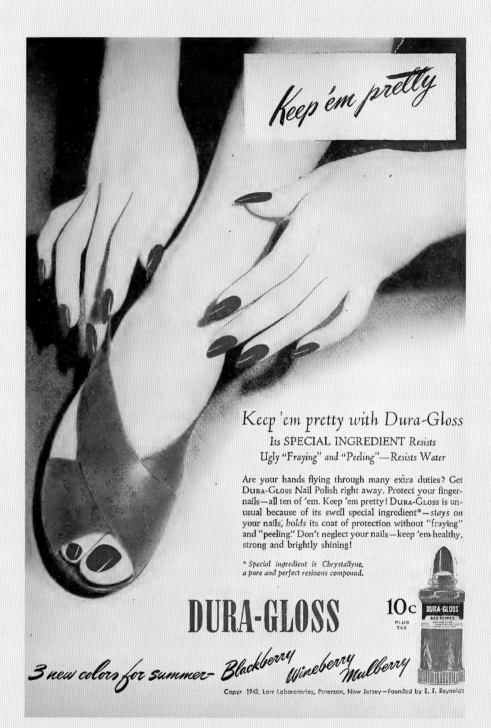

Keep 'em pretty

Keep 'em pretty with Dura-Gloss

Its SPECIAL INGREDIENT Resists
Ugly "Fraying" and "Peeling"—Resists Water

Are your hands flying through many extra duties? Get
Dura-Gloss Nail Polish right away. Protect your fingernails—all ten of 'em. Keep 'em pretty! Dura-Gloss is un-
usual because of its swell special ingredient*—*stays on
your nails, holds its coat of protection without "fraying"
and "peeling." Don't neglect your nails—keep 'em healthy,
strong and brightly shining!

* Special ingredient is Chrystallyne,
a pure and perfect resinous compound.

DURA-GLOSS

10c
PLUS
TAX

3 new colors for summer— Blackberry Wineberry Mulberry

GLAMOUR GIRL'S HOME MANICURE, STEP-BY-STEP

*'I know someone who lost her job because
her nails were such a mess. She was a good actress,
but she simply couldn't get organised when
it came to grooming.'*

– Mitzi Gaynor

YOU WILL NEED:
- Polish remover
- Cuticle remover/cuticle oil
- Flexible emery boards
- Base, polish and topcoat
- Nail brush and a bowl of soap and water
- Cotton balls
- Orange stick
- Nail buffer
- Hand lotion

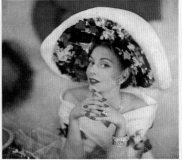

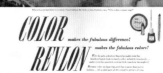

1. Remove every trace of old polish.
2. With your emery board, carefully shape your nails, filing from the outside in. Don't file too close to the outside edges, as this weakens the nail.
3. Spend a few minutes soaking your nails in a bowl of warm, soapy water. Then, give them a good scrub with a soft brush.
4. Never cut your cuticles. Instead, apply a little cuticle oil on a cotton wool ball. Use your orange stick to gently push the cuticle back.
5. Always apply four layers of polish for a rock-hard, long-lasting finish. Start with the base coat; this is what the rest of your polish will cling to. If you've gone for a clear base, so much the better – it

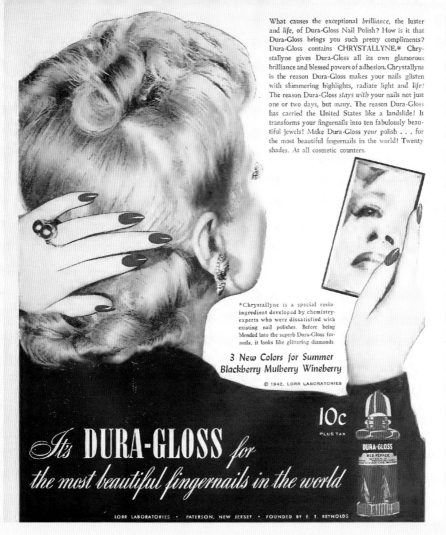

will prevent dark polish from staining the nail bed. Never paint right up to the cuticle and, if you fancy a forties look, leave the very tip of the nail unpainted too – just run your thumb along the tip to remove the excess.

6. Apply two coats of polish. Once these have set, apply a fast-drying, colourless topcoat.
7. Massage your hands with your favourite lotion and enjoy some well-deserved relaxation time.

Top tip! Fake nails aren't just for drama – broken nails can always be replaced with fakes, trimmed and painted to match your own nails. The trick is to make sure the glue is thoroughly dry before you add the polish. Mitzi Gaynor recommends tying the fake on with a piece of string before you go to bed. 'Next morning I put on the polish and that's it,' she says.

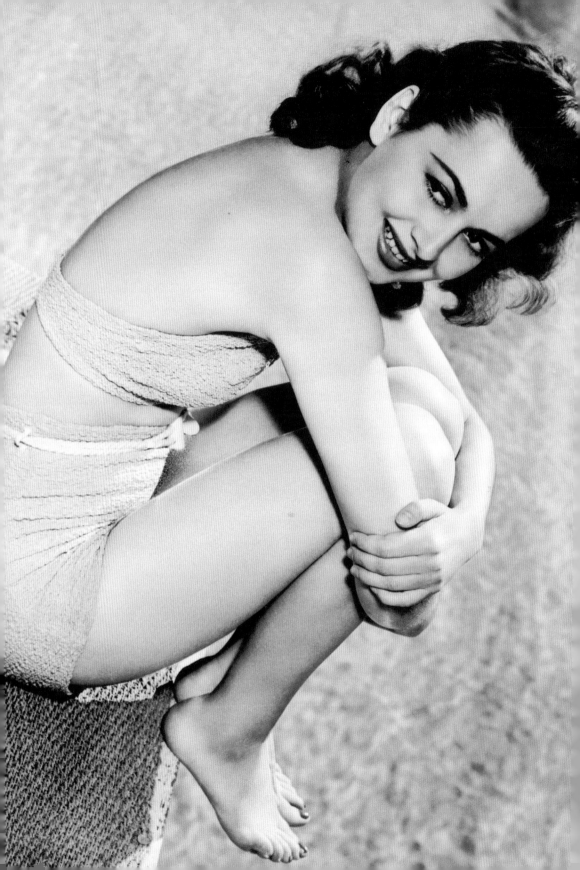

Body Makeup

'A woman's dress should be like a barbed-wire fence: serving its purpose without obstructing the view.'
– Sophia Loren

The silky, slinky gowns of the thirties demanded perfect skin. However lovely the face above the plunging neckline, unsightly spots and tan lines were unforgivable beauty sins, guaranteed to ruin your look. Any would-be glamour girl knew that to use luxurious product on her face, but skimp on body care was a false economy. Can you imagine a screen goddess like Jean Harlow with less than gleaming skin? Of course, the stars knew a few tricks to ensure they were always ready to bare all.

OLIVIA DE HAVILLAND'S ALL-OVER SKIN CARE ROUTINE

1. Using a long-handled brush and plenty of soap, give your back, shoulders and arms a nightly scrub. Don't neglect your elbows, which can get very dry.
2. Apply a little cream afterwards.
3. Once a week – ideally after bathing – give yourself an all-over massage using warm olive oil. Massage into the skin, beginning at your chin and ending at the soles of your feet.
4. Before heading out for the evening, apply a 'makeup blender' to your arms, neck and back in a shade that harmonises with your face powder.

Olivia de Havilland.

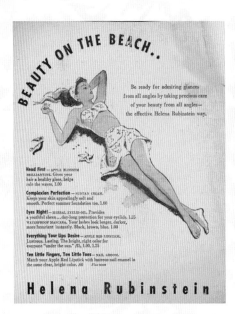

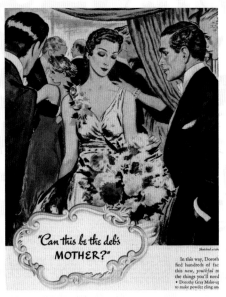

Top tip! Try liquid body makeup for your arms and back – applied with a sponge in a shade that matches the rest of your makeup and won't come off!

SOPHIA LOREN: OLIVE GODDESS

Sixties siren Sophia Loren always insisted that, 'there is a fountain of youth: it is your mind, your talents and the lives of people you love,' but the secret behind her radiant Mediterranean complexion can actually be bought by the bottle. In fact, Sophia owes her age-defying beauty to olive oil. As well as consuming at least two tablespoons of the stuff in her food every day, she'd massage small amounts into her skin (like Olivia). She even made a habit of adding a capful or two to her hot baths. Emma Stone is one modern-day devotee of the moisturising properties of olive oil. 'I have a big bottle on my sink,' the flame-haired starlet recently revealed. 'It makes my skin smell like focaccia.'

Sophia Loren.

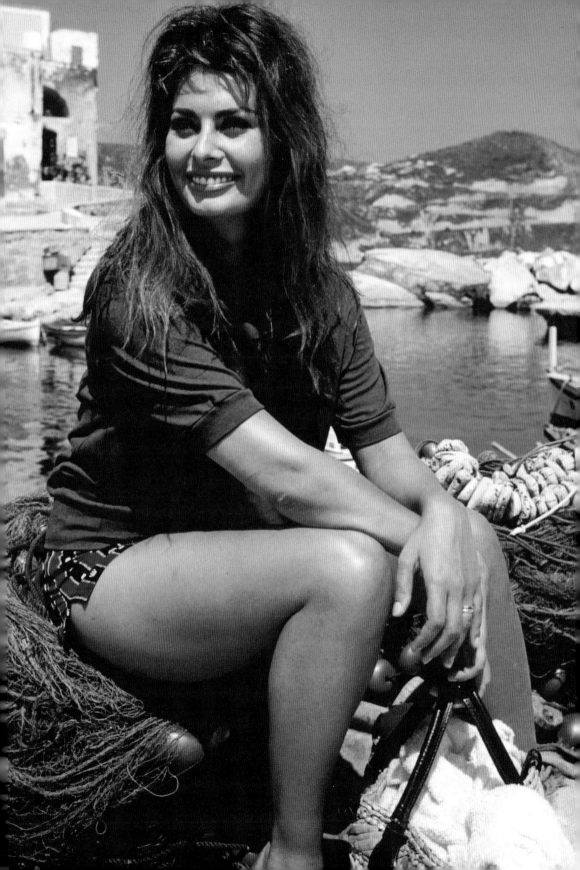

DÉCOLLETAGE MAKEUP TO DAZZLE

When wearing a low-cut dress, daring décolletage makeup is a must. Beauty advisers will tell you that any shade applied to this area needs to blend seamlessly with the rest of your makeup. Even so, Greta Garbo famously ignored this rule, dusting her décolletage with a sparkling, reflective powder that was several enchanting shades lighter than what she was wearing on her face. Another clever trick, developed by Perc Westmore for Carole Lombard in 1934's *Lady by Choice* (at Carole's request), helped the actress to make the most of her natural assets. Here's how he achieved the fuller look:

1. Highlight across your chest and décolletage with lightweight, liquid foundation, followed by powder.
2. Top with a little cold cream or Vaseline for extra emphasis.
3. To finish, run a thin line of powdered rouge (*not* cream or liquid) down the inside of the cleavage.

Left: *Marlene Dietrich*. Right: *Dorothy Lamour*.

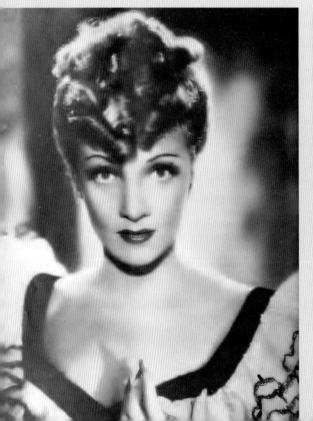
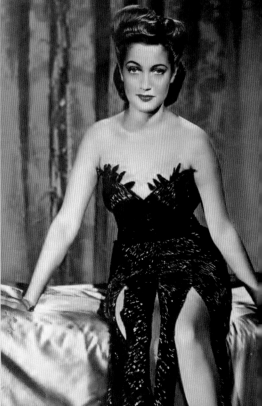

Vintage Inspiration: Seventy years later, the crew behind *Pirates of the Caribbean* used this trick to transform slender Keira Knightley into corset-bound beauty Elizabeth Swann. 'They painted my breasts on for the films, which is extraordinary because it's kind of a dying art form,' Keira revealed of the 45-minute process. 'And I completely loved it . . . I didn't even need surgery.'

PERFECT PERFUME

'I love perfume. I never go without it. In fact, I have gone without other things to buy it.'
– Audrey Hepburn

Like most girls, I never feel really made up and ready to go for the evening without a spritz of perfume. Here's how to make the most of your favourite scents.

- Wear appropriately. Warner Bros. starlet Joan Leslie recommends swapping your usual scent for a little eau de Cologne to give you a faintly alluring smell without seeming inappropriately flashy at work.
- Luxuriate. 'To some people, a bath is just a bath – but it should be more,' says Fay Wray. 'Stimulating perfumes inspire people to be beautiful.' Try adding scented oils to make your time in the tub more pleasurable.
- Combine. Lucille Ball always wore two scents: eau de Cologne, rubbed into her skin after bathing, and then perfume, added after dressing.
- Don't let your perfume take over. 'Subtlety, that's what men like,' says Marilyn Monroe. 'I believe they don't like to be so overwhelmed by perfume that instead of thinking of you, they are thinking, "What is she wearing?"'
- Make it personal. Another Marilyn rule is to find a fragrance that is 'not too popular' and dab on small amounts all over your body.

'I rarely use it on my clothes, but when I start to dress I spray it on my knees and all the way up to my eyebrows so that the fragrance really belongs to me,' she confides.

'Once upon a time there were perfumes that didn't smell like candy and sweetness. I mean, Marlene Dietrich would not have worn a perfume that had vanilla in it. Some of my favourite perfumes are Quelques Fleurs and Lancôme Magie Noire. Jean Paul Gaultier Classique is also so nice; it smells like makeup.'
– Dita Von Teese

THE FIRST CELEBRITY SCENT

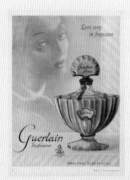

Audrey Hepburn went one better than 'not too popular' in 1957 – when her close personal friend and trusted *couturier* Hubert de Givenchy designed a new fragrance especially for her. Audrey was the only woman to wear 'L'interdit' for a full year before the flowery scent was released. It was Givenchy's first perfume, but not – as some claim – the first celebrity-endorsed fragrance. Back in 1930, 29-year-old silent film star Lila Lee promoted the inappropriately-named 'Seventeen', in ads that claimed 'a perfume . . . taught me the secret of youth'.

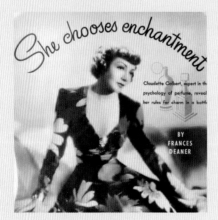

Top tip! Mae West recommends rubbing a little of your most delicate scent into the palm of your hand, before smoothing your husband's weary brow. 'It's a safe bet he won't go out that night!' says Mae.

Marilyn Monroe.

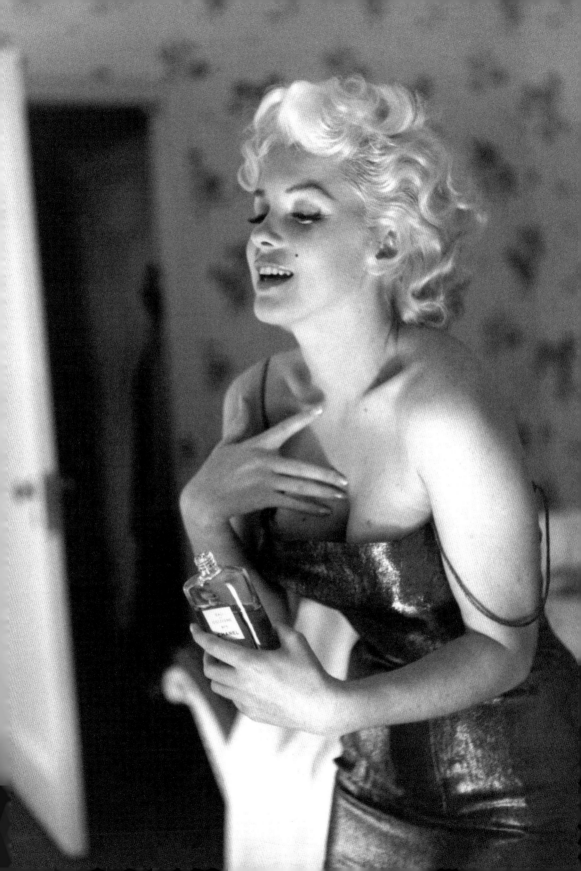

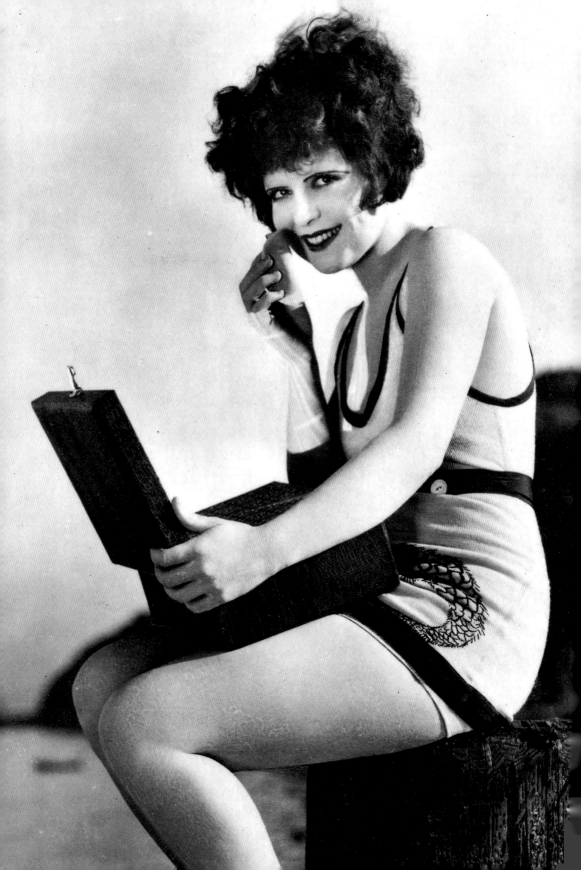

Get the Look

CLARA BOW'S IT GIRL CHARM

Although Clara herself preferred a golden tan, her pallid on-screen persona was always well-powdered, with a perfect Cupid's bow and lashings of smoky kohl liner. It was this style that girls on the street chose to copy. Here's how you can too:

1. After your usual foundation, apply a generous dusting of powder – as pale as you can get away with.
2. Follow this up with a minimal amount of rouge, worn high to keep from emphasising round faces like Clara's.
3. Apply plenty of kohl to the upper and lower lash lines. Don't be afraid to extend beyond the outer edges of your eyes – this will give you Clara's elongated look – and blend with your finger for a smoky effect.
4. Darken the lashes with mascara – fake lashes, a new concept, were popular during this period but Clara didn't need them.
5. Apply a light shadow to your lids and blend with a little baby oil. This wet look was popular as it reflected back the studio lights – even if it was one of Max Factor's pet hates!
6. Clara's brows were shaved off and drawn back on, '20s style. But you can simply cover yours up with wax or concealer.

Clara Bow.

Clara Bow wearing 'Maybelline mascara'

You, too, can have **EYES** *that* **Charm!**

A touch of "MAYBELLINE" works beauty wonders. Even light, scant eyelashes are made to appear naturally dark, long and luxurious. All the hidden loveliness of your eyes, their brilliance, depth and expression—is instantly revealed. The difference is remarkable. Millions of women in all parts of the world, even the most beautiful actresses of the stage and screen, now realise that "MAYBELLINE" is the most important aid to beauty and use it regularly. Perfectly harmless in every way.

Sold at your good Drug & Department Store, etc.

Maybelline
Eyelash Beautifier

7. Using a heavy black pencil, draw two new lines straight across your brow, dipping sharply down when you reach the end of the brow bone.
8. Choose a shade of red lipstick to match the flapper's daring personality (Clara once said she was 'defined by vermilion') and draw into a Cupid's bow. Make sure you powder over your lips first to hide their natural contours. Finish with a second dusting of powder to prevent smudging.
9. Add a heart-shaped beauty spot to reflect Clara's peppy sense of fun.
10. Finish with rose-pink nail varnish (Clara's favourite), painted onto neatly filed nails. Combine with a twenties-style windswept bob and you're good to go!

Fabulous flappers: Carey Mulligan's turn as Daisy Buchanan in *The Great Gatsby* (2013) provides a master class in how to rock vintage style with a contemporary twist. Despite adhering to the basic demands of the

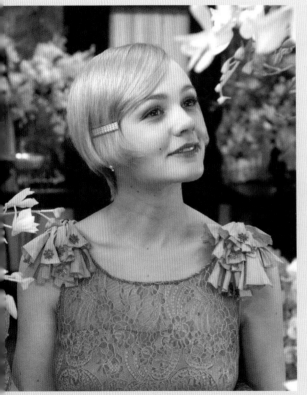

era – 'the eyebrows were the most important part of the face because they represented the fashion of the time,' revealed Maurizio Silvi, the makeup artist who masterminded Carey's twenties transformation – Silvi was unafraid to experiment with the flapper's signature look. 'We decided that red lipstick didn't fit Daisy's personality,' Silvi explained. Instead, Carey's lips were slicked with a shimmery nude shade (Chanel Rouge Allure in Séduisante) – ensuring that even in a crowd of crimson-lipped society vixens, Daisy was the one to catch the eye of dashing Jay Gatsby. Topped off with a charming black beauty spot, the end result is a spellbinding update on the twenties trend.

Carey Mulligan.

JEAN HARLOW'S BOMBSHELL BEAUTY

Atrue glamour goddess, everything about Jean Harlow shimmered: from her impossibly blonde locks to her satin evening gowns. Her house was decorated throughout in white, gilt and marble, and MGM even did up her dressing room to match her hair. Throughout the thirties, her influence was enormous; inspiring women everywhere to bleach their hair and faces – all of them desperate to look like Jean . . . though no one shone quite so bright.

1. Apply primer and crème foundation to give you the best possible coverage. Layer on concealer wherever you need a little extra help (under the eyes, for instance), since Jean's ethereal look demands a flawless complexion. 'Very few people who admire blonde hair realise that every little speck of dust or grime appears on the surface as . . . on a white dress or coat,' Jean herself once sighed. Even so, her shimmery perfection is well worth the effort!

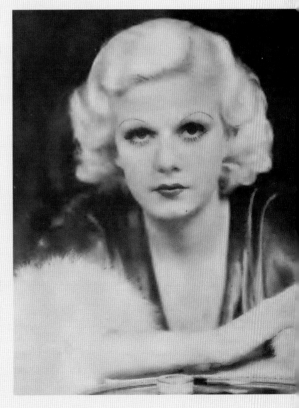

2. Delicate half-moon brows were Jean's sweet-and-sultry trademark, so pencil yours in high, narrow arches. Jean shaved her natural brows off altogether and drew them back in with a 'finely-pointed pencil' (as revealed by *Photoplay* in 1933), but you can always disguise rather than remove your brows using concealer or wax. Don't be afraid to sweep down past your brow bone at the outer corners to frame your pretty eyes.

Jean Harlow.

3. Select a duo of complementary eye shadows to match your colouring. Jean often opted for shades of blue to match her on-trend navy mascara. To get her dreamy, deep-set gaze, dust your creases with the darker shadow. Next brush your lids with the shimmery lighter shade and blend together – perfect for those 'come hither' glances!

4. Recreate Jean's long, dark lashes with fakes on both your top and bottom eyelids. Apply mascara over the top to blend with your natural lashes.

Beauty Shop — Conducted By Carolyn Van Wyck

All the beauty tricks of all the stars brought to you each month

HIGH, narrow and very arched are Jean's eyebrows. She uses a finely pointed eyebrow pencil. The high brow enlarges the eye, gives clarity, an appealing quality.

JEAN uses a true red cream rouge for her lips, blending the line perfectly and carrying the color well inside to prevent a break in tone. Those very long lashes are black.

SKIN-TONE powder is then puffed lightly but thoroughly over Jean's face and neck, with special attention to nostrils, eye corners and chin. And, always brush from brows.

JEAN'S platinum halo has probably aroused more comment and curiosity than any one feature of any star. Naturally blonde, Jean encourages whiteness by weekly shampoos with white soap and a final rinse containing a few drops of French bluing. She brushes for softness, sets her wave with water and vinegar.

5. To get Jean's trademark 'bracket lips', powder over the natural contours of your lips. Create your new lip line with a bold red pencil. Bracket lips are all about curves, so make sure your line bows from the corner of your mouth up to the first peak, has a deep swoop down in the centre (dipping below the natural lip line if necessary) and curves again as you come down to the opposite corner. The lower lip should be significantly smaller than the upper.

6. Fill in the lines with a strong red lipstick that has plenty of gloss (this is not the time for matte), focusing on the centre of the mouth especially.

7. Finish with a generous dusting of powder and a beauty spot, drawn on with eyebrow pencil. Jean's moved about from her chin to the corner of her mouth, but the effect was always dazzling.

Top tip! For a true Harlow effect, ensure your habiliment is perfectly chosen to set off your style. Divinely pale Jean liked to wear black evening gowns for maximum impact.

Modern-day bombshell: Channelling Jean Harlow is no mean feat. But No Doubt songstress Gwen Stefani pulled it off with aplomb in 2004's

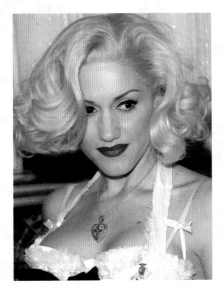

The Aviator. For her shimmery, blonde cameo, Gwen's makeup artist added radiance to her already glowing skin (like Marlene Dietrich, Gwen swears by baby oil as a source of constant moisture) with YSL's Touche Éclat highlighter stick. On stage with her band, Gwen has flirted with a colourful array of bindis and smoky eye makeup to add an extra element to her devastating retro style. One staple she'll never tire of, however, is her show-stopping Ruby Woo lipstick by MAC.

Gwen Stefani.

GRETA GARBO'S MYSTERIOUS MAGNETISM

'The aim of good makeup is not to look like makeup, so be sure the powder exactly matches the colour of your skin.'
– Greta Garbo

In the opulent thirties, Greta's look was startlingly understated. She cleverly concentrated her makeup on her striking eyes and lips. She wore very little on the rest of her face and kept her hair, clothing and jewellery equally simple. Slacks and turtle-necks formed the staples of Greta's wardrobe, and her favourite colours were black, white and grey – all of which exaggerated her ethereal paleness.

1. Greta's skin had a natural glow of its own, so the base for this look

– luminous, light-reflecting primer, topped with liquid foundation and just a dusting of powder – should be as light as you can get away with. Greta applied a pale shade of 'rice powder' – a very light, soft variety of powder – using a chamois rather than a puff. Remember that the spirit of her style is unadorned and minimalist, so if you don't happen to be a Swedish sylph, it's better to substitute white for a shade that suits you personally.

2. Apply a tiny amount of rouge, following the natural line of colour in your cheeks.

3. Eyebrows should be plucked very thin and high, and filled in with eye pencil. If you prefer, you can shave them off and draw them back, but pencilled-on brows should be slightly thicker than the twenties style.

4. Lightly outline your eyes in a shade that suits you. Blonde Greta usually opted for brown, but brunettes may achieve a more striking effect with black.

5. Dust your creases with a dark, smoky shade to make your eyes appear deeper and more mysterious. Remember that the arch of the eyebrow, the curve of the eye socket and the contour of the eye should all harmonise.

6. Fake lashes, trimmed to fit, create a fuller, more natural look. Greta had wispy, blonde lashes and applied a huge quantity of fakes to frame her eyes – each one made of real hair and painstakingly applied with tweezers and lash-destroying spirit gum. Today, you could probably use a volumising mascara to achieve the same effect with much less hassle. Apply to top and bottom lashes and be sure to add a little extra to the outer lashes to accentuate the almond shape of your eyes.

7. Apply a natural shade of lipstick for the daytime, choosing a more striking colour for evenings. Greta herself liked dark red shades. Lips should be drawn fairly straight, but never exaggeratedly small or thin. Apply lipstick thoroughly on the lower lip, but add very little to the upper.

8. Go for a very simple hairstyle so as not to distract from your meticulously made-up face. Greta's favourite was a long bob, parted to one side and swept back from her brow. The look was invented for her by the inimitable Monsieur Antoine (otherwise

Greta Garbo.

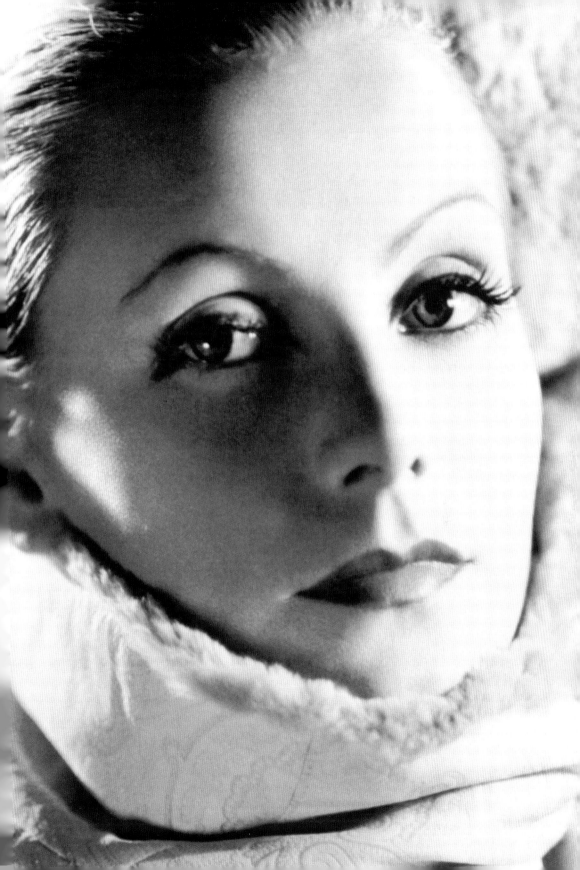

known as celebrity hairdresser Antoni Cierplikowski) and she stuck to it for most of her life.

9. Dress plainly; accessorise simply. Greta favoured pretty pearls and onyx jewellery to match her black, white and grey wardrobe. On formal occasions, she'd wear white orchids and narcissi – as exotic adornments that complemented her natural beauty perfectly.

Timeless tip: Lining the eye socket with eyeliner (rather than a darker shade of shadow) was a striking trend that would regain popularity in the 1960s. Compare Greta's look with Audrey Hepburn's to see how vintage styles can be updated and incorporated into more modern looks.

1930S GOLDEN GIRLS

'Glamour is what I sell. It's my stock in trade.'
– Marlene Dietrich

Like the Depression never happened, the movie goddesses of the thirties embraced gilded glamour in a big way. Rumour has it that decadent Marlene Dietrich insisted on her wigs being dusted with real gold. From shimmering evening gowns – skin-tight and dripping with sequins and beads – to burnished golden hair, gold eye shadow and lacquered lips, the thirties look is all about luxurious indulgence. For wannabe golden girls, the essentials are as follows:

• Shimmery powder to finish (rather than real gold à la Dietrich). You can go for luminous white or healthy bronze, but either way you'll shine.
• Metallic eye shadow (gold, silver or bronze) used alone or combined with other shades. A metallic overcoat will give your lids that beautiful thirties lustre. Brunettes and dark redheads should try mahogany shadow (applied first) topped with gold: the deep colour will exaggerate the size of your eyes, while the gold flecks are guaranteed to dazzle. For blondes, combine royal blue with silver; Ann Vernon swears, 'it will make even a strong man's heart thump alarmingly'.

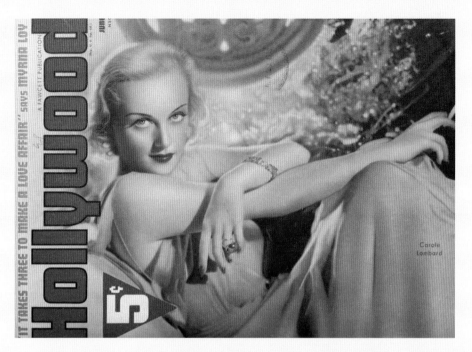

Carole Lombard

- Try tipping your lashes with gold or silver. Wait for your regular mascara to dry and then apply a little metallic shadow to the tips – this may stick better if you apply a little Vaseline first.
- Glossy metallic lipstick, slicked on for a shiny, lacquered look – applied over another deeper colour or alone. Sheer lipsticks (Lipstick Queen's Butterfly Ball range, for example) are especially good for adding just a subtle sheen.
- Gilded nails. You could even try combining more than one metallic shade. Start with a golden base coat and follow up with silver over the top for a truly shimmering effect.
- Smooth, glossy locks. Curls and waves should be sculpted rather than undone.
- Opulent ornaments: feathers, gold leaves, sequinned caps, glinting veils, and – of course – flashy jewellery are all features of this most luxurious look. Nail ornaments can also be worn; try adding little butterflies and flowers (like the kind you get in confetti) before applying your top coat of clear gloss.

Modern-day master class: When it comes to glowing thirties-inspired glamour, Beyoncé Knowles is queen. Here's a list of essential products

– taken out on the road by her trusted makeup artist Sir John – to keep her shining like a diva.

- For sleep-deprived skin, the songstress' 'go-to product' is Caudalie's Beauty Elixir. You can achieve a similarly dewy look by adding a drop or two of illuminator to your favourite moisturising oil.
- Metallic eye shadow to emphasise stunning almond eyes. Even if you're not inclined to go full-beam – coating your entire lid with colour – Sir John suggests you, 'try adding a copper, silver or bronze to the inner-corners (tear ducts) . . . which is always quite charming to gaze upon.'
- Super shiny lip-gloss – not just for lips, but to slick on over your eye makeup. Sir John recommends, 'just a tiny amount. You're not trying to coat it like you would your lips. You just want to give lustre to the eye so it reflects light.' Begin with a base of waterproof shadow and prepare to lighten up beautifully. As mentioned, Marlene Dietrich was working similar wonders with baby oil decades earlier . . .

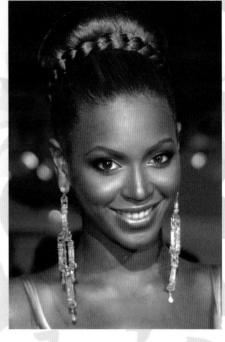

Beyoncé Knowles.

PIN-UP GIRLS

'This is a strictly work-a-day world.
For that reason, romance and gaiety begin
for most of us in the evening . . . That is when we
transform ourselves from practical, hard-working girls
into glamorous and alluring creatures!'
– Ann Vernon

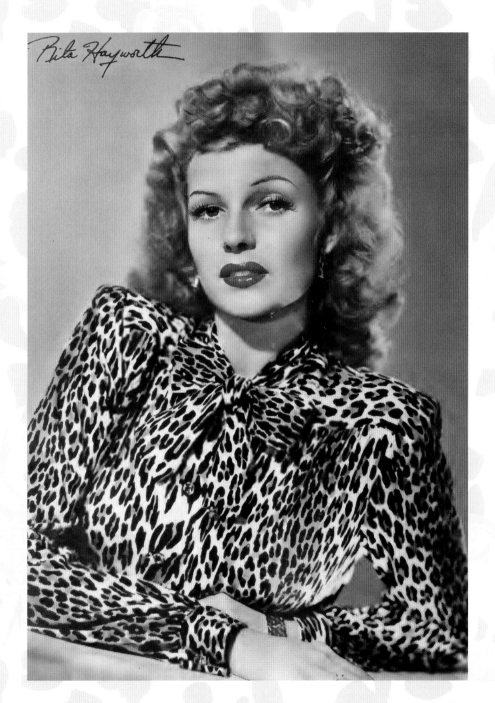

Rita Hayworth.

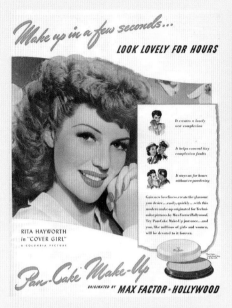
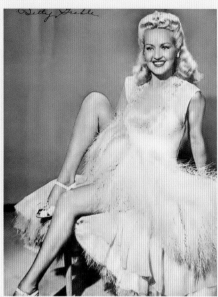

Left: *Rita Hayworth*. Right: *Betty Grable*.

Back in the forties, sirens like Rita Hayworth, Betty Grable and Dorothy Lamour certainly did their bit for the war effort, selling war bonds, touring service camps and more. Most of all, these girls boosted morale, giving servicemen something to fight for and reminding everyone else of the meaning of glamour. Pin-up girls were ultra-feminine beauties: their hair and nails were long, their clothes just revealing enough and their lips painted with 'victory red'.

1. Start with a natural foundation with a rosy tint and apply a rosy powder on top. In the evening, try applying a *very* light layer of blusher all over your face; the hint of pink will counteract the effect of harsh electric lighting on your night out.
2. Carefully outline your lips with colour and a fine brush, starting in the centre and working out. Draw slightly over your natural lip-line if necessary to create a full, heart-shaped pout.
3. Fill in the lips with a matching shade of red making sure they are really well covered in the centre. Try Liz Taylor's trick of dusting the lips with finishing powder before applying a second coat and blot well.
4. Apply eye shadow in a natural colour that harmonises with your

eyes – blue, blue-grey, grey, green, brown and violet were the most popular shades of the forties. Apply evenly over the lid but never above the curve of your eye socket. Remember, the forties look is all about the lips, so don't let your eyes dominate.

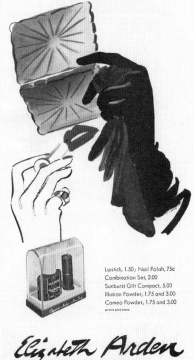

Lipstick, 1.50; Nail Polish, 75c
Combination Set, 2.00
Sunburst Gilt Compact, 5.00
Illusion Powder, 1.75 and 3.00
Cameo Powder, 1.75 and 3.00
prices plus taxes

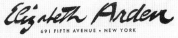

691 FIFTH AVENUE • NEW YORK

5. Apply a line of liquid liner close to the top lashes. Widen slightly at the outer corner of the eye and extend a little beyond the lid to create an exaggerated almond shape.

6. Brush eyebrows up and out; then pluck from below, following the natural curve of your brow. Don't make them too thin. If you're heading out for the evening, brush on a little baby oil to add gloss and keep them tidy.

7. Go with natural eyelashes for a true forties look – fakes were hard to come by in wartime. The fashion was to apply mascara painstakingly one lash at a time with a tiny brush and cake mascara if you had it (burnt cork if you didn't), allowing each lash to dry before moving on to the next. However you choose to recreate this effect, be sure to ply the eyelash curler with enthusiasm beforehand – so as to give your lashes a dramatic, eye-opening 'swoop'.

8. Match your nail colour to your lips – exactly if you can – and wear them long. Be sure to apply a double coat of colour followed by a top coat for added gloss.

9. Brush hair back from the brow to exaggerate the length of the face.

10. Neat and tidy was very much the order of the day, so be sure to fix any curls and waves in place with a heavy-duty hair spray. Alternatively, tie them up in a stylish headscarf.

Modern-day master class: Dita Von Teese's snow-white complexion demands a classic red lip. Unwilling to start her day without a swipe of the stuff – 'I've always loved that statement of colour on my face,' the burlesque beauty revealed – Dita's passion for red is verging on obsession. As well as hoarding vintage lipstick tubes, she admits to filling them with frozen modern product. YSL Rouge Pur Couture Glossy Stain in Rose Tempura 13 and Dior Roulette Red are two of her most coveted shades. 'Everyone always thinks I'm so done up,' she confided, 'but it's just the lipstick!' As for the secret to making your colour last: Dita advises a matte finish rather than gloss. 'Powdery red looks so beautiful and lasts longer than everything else.'

SOPHIA LOREN'S SIREN STYLE

'Being beautiful is no handicap so long
as you don't think too much about it.'
– Sophia Loren

Sophia Loren has one of the most striking faces ever to grace the screen, but her beauty is far from conventional and didn't instantly enchant *everyone* in Tinseltown. 'After every screen test it was the same story from the technicians,' she writes in *Women & Beauty*. '"There is no way to make this girl look good – her nose is too long and her hips are too broad." And would I think about trimming off just a bit of my nose?' But rather than give in to pressure to go under the knife, feisty Sophia made a conscious decision to spotlight her best feature: her eyes. And when you have eyes like this sexy signorina (not to mention her fabulous hourglass figure), you have some promising material to work with. Armed with lashings of smouldering black kohl, Sophia created a look that was both highly alluring and highly individual – making her one of the most copied stars of the fifties and sixties. She once said she wasn't the girl-next-door; she was the girl men *wished* lived next door.

1. Even when she chose to go bare-faced, Sophia's olive skin had a sun-kissed glow of its own. If you're blessed with a similarly gorgeous

Sophia Loren.

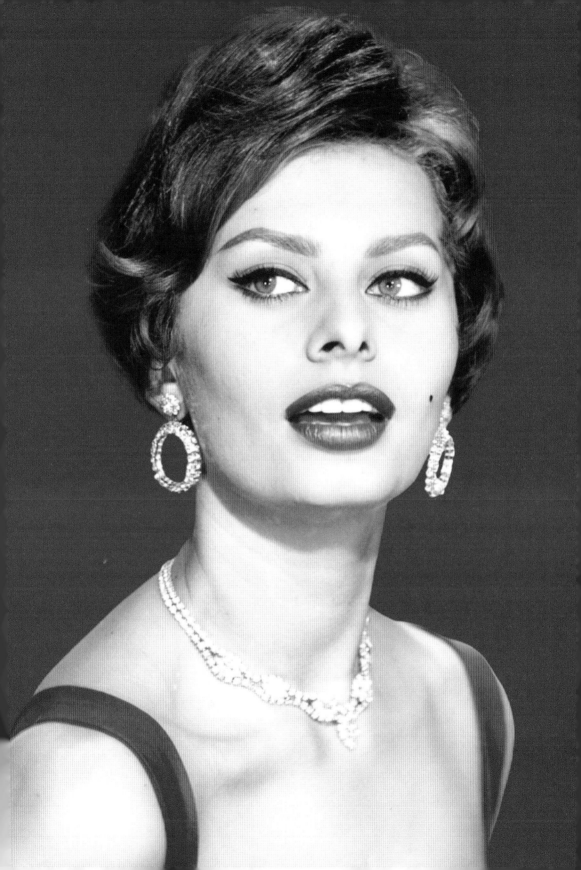

Mediterranean complexion, all you need to set it off is a little bronzing powder dusted over a peach or beige-based foundation. If you're naturally pale, try adding warmth with a crème foundation that's a shade or two darker than you'd usually wear – just don't forget to blend down below your jawline for seamless coverage.

2. Apply rouge to your cheekbones, sweeping back towards your temples. Avoid the hollows of your cheeks. Sophia used an orange-based rouge to match the warm undertone of her skin.

3. Sophia shaved her eyebrows and drew them back on using painstaking individual strokes in a mixture of black and beige pencil. If you don't fancy removing your brows altogether (or bleaching them, which was another of Sophia's beauty tricks), you can still achieve her look by careful shaping and colouring. Sophia's eyebrows were often quite angular; so keep yours straight at both ends with a bow in the middle. They should also arch a little beyond the brow bone, emphasising the slant of the eyes below.

4. Sophia's famous 'cat's eyes' also had a strong upward slant, which you can create with a black gel liner – in the form of a pen or a pot and brush combo. Start with a fine line along the upper lashes, drawn with your pen or brush. It should stretch to the outer edge of the eye, going up slightly as you pass the outer corner of the eye. Starting at the middle of the lash line, trace over your original line, building up the slant, until you have achieved Sophia's dramatic almond shape.

5. Draw along the lower lash line, starting just short of the tear duct and curving up towards the outer corner of the eye. This lower line should follow the curve of the upper line, joining up with it at the outer corners.

6. Sophia's lashes were equally ample, so use curlers to help you achieve her impressive sweep. Next, apply a good layer of mascara to the top lashes, doubling up at the outer corners. Use a little less on the lower lashes.

7. Sophia's lipstick follows the natural shape of her lips, but with exaggerated curves. She especially liked to emphasise the cleft in the middle. She had naturally full lips, so you may need to go slightly over your natural lip line to achieve her look. Outline the lips with pencil first and, when you're happy with the shape, fill them in with a good matte lipstick. Sophia tended to wear beige or orange lipstick during the day and orange-based reds in the

evening. Again, these were colours that complemented her sultry olive skin tone.

8. Draw a perfectly rounded beauty spot on one cheekbone for added va-va-voom. This also served to draw attention to Sophia's fantastic bone structure.

Wear this strong makeup with big hair and striking clothing – Sophia herself liked red, which she considered 'the colour of life.'

Modern-day master class: Like Sophia Loren before her, Penelope Cruz's signature look is fresh-faced. Her glowing olive skin requires only the lightest coat of Chanel's Teint Innocence Foundation (in Soft Honey) – just don't expect to see her soulful brown eyes adorned with anything less than lashings of mascara and kohl liner. 'Mascara is the little black dress for your eyes,' she once quipped.

Penelope Cruz.

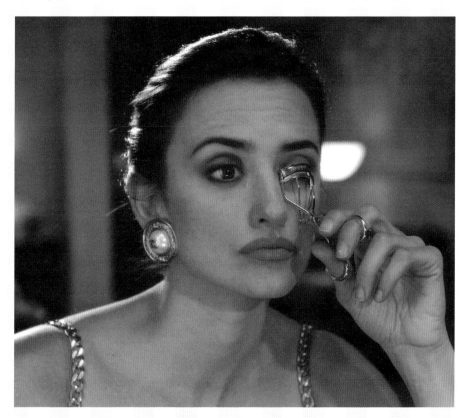

MARILYN'S BLONDE-ALL-OVER GLOW

'I'm personally opposed to a deep tan
because I like to feel blonde all over.'
– Marilyn Monroe

With her luminous complexion, tousled curls and ruby lips, what girl hasn't wished she could recreate just a little of Marilyn's magic at home? Despite her shimmering bombshell looks, Marilyn was no dumb blonde. 'Study your face carefully to decide what features you want to focus attention on,' she once advised. 'No man likes a girl whose face looks like a piece of fancily decorated pastry, but if you're careful you can even bring up the heavy guns like eye shadow and he'll never know you're "made-up" at all! In my view most girls look more desirable with glistening lids and a moist mouth. A drop of oil on the lids will give the effect and if you're handy with a lipstick brush there's nothing like it for that luscious look.' Though she never gave away any more specific secrets than these, there's been endless speculation about the products and techniques she used to achieve her gorgeous 'blonde-all-over glow'. Here's how she might have gone about it had she had modern products at her perfectly-manicured fingertips.

1. Celebrity photographer Eve Arnold never quite got over the beauty of Marilyn's pearly white skin. And that's the base you'll need to achieve her look. Marilyn herself applied a combination of Vaseline, hormone cream and Erno Laszlo's Active Phelityl Cream to give her skin its trademark lustre under the studio lights. Thankfully, you can create the same dewy sheen by prepping your skin with luminous primer. Filled with light-reflecting pigments, That Gal by Benefit provides a modern-day shortcut to Marilyn's complexion.

2. Apply a medium-coverage foundation in as pale a tone as you can wear. Even if you prefer matte, you'll want to opt for something with a dewy finish. Top with a generous dusting of powder that's just a shade darker than your foundation. If your chosen product includes a little shimmer, so much the better. Adding a subtle,

stardust-like finish, Guerlain's Meteorite Pearls are perfect for this look. This will give your skin Marilyn's captivating 'white-showing-through' look.

3. Complete with a touch of coral rouge dusted along your cheekbones.
4. Highlight below your brows, around the outer corners of your

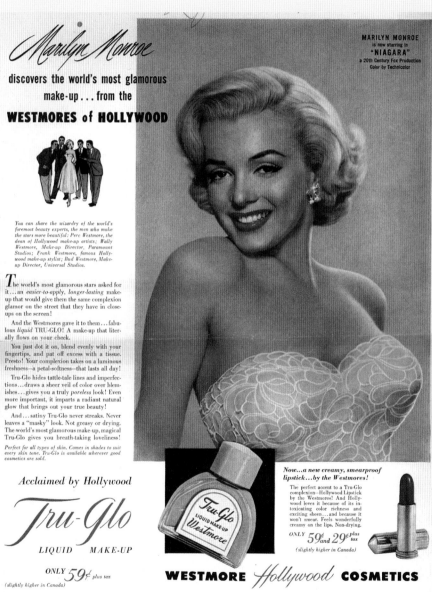

Marilyn Monroe

discovers the world's most glamorous make-up...from the

WESTMORES of HOLLYWOOD

You can share the wizardry of the world's foremost beauty experts, the men who make the stars more beautiful; Perc Westmore, the dean of Hollywood make-up artists; Wally Westmore, Make-up Director, Paramount Studios; Frank Westmore, famous Hollywood make-up stylist; Bud Westmore, Make-up Director, Universal Studios.

The world's most glamorous stars asked for it...an *easier-to-apply, longer-lasting* make-up that would give them the same complexion glamor on the street that they have in close-ups on the screen!

And the Westmores gave it to them...fabulous *liquid* TRU-GLO! A make-up that literally flows on your cheek.

You just dot it on, blend evenly with your fingertips, and pat off excess with a tissue. Presto! Your complexion takes on a luminous freshness—a petal-softness—that lasts all day!

Tru-Glo hides tattle-tale lines and imperfections...draws a sheer veil of color over blemishes...gives you a truly *poreless* look! Even more important, it imparts a radiant natural glow that brings out your true beauty!

And...satiny Tru-Glo never streaks. Never leaves a "masky" look. Not greasy or drying. The world's most glamorous make-up, magical Tru-Glo gives you breath-taking loveliness!

Perfect for all types of skin. Comes in shades to suit every skin tone. Tru-Glo is available wherever good cosmetics are sold.

Acclaimed by Hollywood

Tru-Glo

LIQUID   MAKE-UP

ONLY 59¢ *plus tax*

(slightly higher in Canada)

Now...a new creamy, smearproof lipstick...by the Westmores!

The perfect accent to a Tru-Glo complexion—Hollywood Lipstick by the Westmores! And Hollywood loves it because of its intoxicating color richness and exciting sheen...and because it won't smear. Feels wonderfully creamy on the lips. Non-drying.

ONLY 59¢ *and* 29¢ *plus tax*

(slightly higher in Canada)

WESTMORE *Hollywood* **COSMETICS**

eyes and anywhere else you need a little extra sheen using a luminescent product like Stila's All Over Shimmer – a trick that never failed to spotlight Marilyn's beautiful blue eyes.

5. Marilyn's eye shadow was in subtle harmony with her colouring, so dust your lids with a neutral shade that suits. Marilyn herself opted for pale pink or cool brown taupe, blended with a slightly darker tint along the crease of her socket; this made her eyes look deeper-set. Bobbi Brown's shimmer brick in various shades of beige should help you achieve this three-dimensional look. Like Clara Bow, Marilyn topped her shadow with a tiny drop of oil to make her lids 'glisten invitingly'.

6. Apply liquid liner to your upper lash line, sticking as close to the lashes as possible. Depending on whether she was going for a subtle daytime look or full-on evening glam, Marilyn would alternate between brown and black, possibly teamed with a second, barely-there line of gold running just above. Taper the line from thin to thick (towards the middle) to thin again, extending out beyond the corner of your eye in a subtle flick.

7. Marilyn's makeup artist Allan 'Whitey' Snyder also lined the rim, or waterline, of her lower lid with white eye pencil, extending the line out beyond the edge of her eye to mirror the flick of the line on top. This trick made Marilyn's naturally lovely eyes appear wider.

8. Take a pair of strip-lashes and cut one of them in two. Apply one customised half-lash to each eye, so that it covers from the middle of your lid to the outer corner. Creating the illusion of curly lashes that flick out at the side, this is sure to give you Marilyn's seductive, half-closed look.

9. When shaping your brows, keep them thick but tapering slightly away at either end. Pluck them in arches that mirror the curve of your lips and shade with a pencil that matches your natural colouring.

10. Marilyn's lips are drawn in an amped-up version of the classic Cupid's bow (as worn by her idol, Jean Harlow). Marilyn's style is squarer at the bottom with high curves in the middle, slanting steeply down towards the corners of her mouth. The colour, of course, is red for glamour (although Marilyn herself preferred pink for everyday wear).

11. To achieve a captivating, multi-dimensional look, Marilyn slicked

Marilyn Monroe.

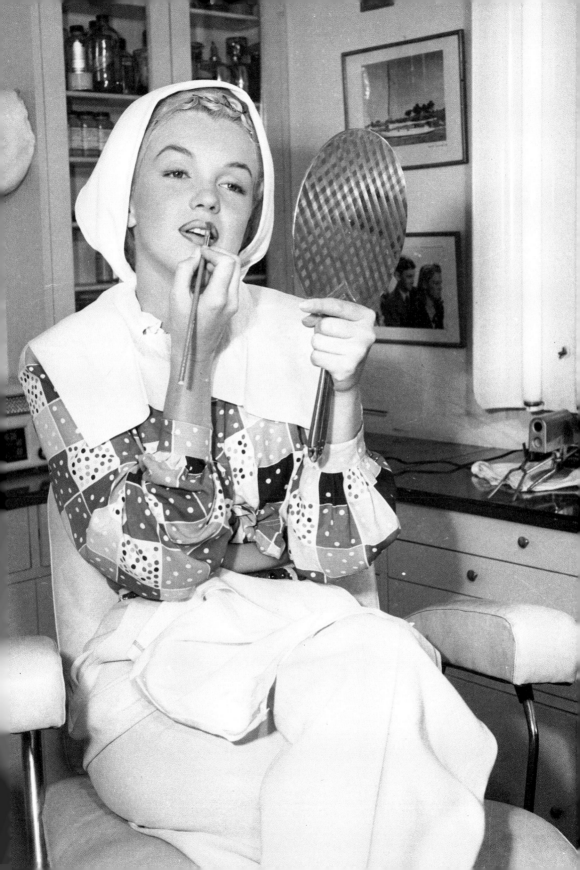

on up to five different shades of lipstick, saving darker reds for the outer-edges of her lips. Like Marilyn, you can use more eye-catching glossy shades to draw attention to the centre of your pout. She also added white dewy highlights above her Cupid's bow and below her pillowy bottom lip. She topped her lips with a gloss mixture of her own making – mostly Vaseline.

Marilyn finished off her look with 'a kind of modified pageboy' hairstyle she designed herself. Notice how the curls below the jaw and height on top add length. By brushing her hair back to expose her widow's peak, she cleverly emphasises her heart-shaped face.

Warning! A side-effect of Marilyn's beauty regime was excess facial hair caused by the hormone cream she used. The studio wanted Marilyn to shave it off, but she refused, saying that she liked the way the lights caught the peachy down on her cheeks, making them glow.

ELIZABETH TAYLOR'S
EGYPTIAN ALLURE

'Cleopatra was the most chaotic time in my life, what with le scandale, the Vatican banning me, people making threats on my life, falling madly in love . . . oceans of tears, but some good times too.'
– Elizabeth Taylor

Thanks to her sultry turn as Cleopatra back in 1963, Elizabeth Taylor will always be synonymous with the Queen of the Nile. As well as igniting her romance with swarthy leading man Richard Burton, Elizabeth's spellbinding winged eyes inspired a mania for Egyptian-inspired chic. 'If looks could kill this one will!' promised a sensational ad by Revlon in 1962. Featuring a dusky-eyed temptress

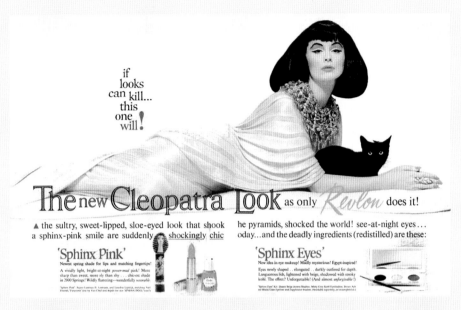

if
looks
can kill...
this
one
will!

The new Cleopatra Look as only *Revlon* does it!

▲ the sultry, sweet-lipped, sloe-eyed look that shook a sphinx-pink smile are suddenly and shockingly chic

he pyramids, shocked the world! see-at-night eyes... oday...and the deadly ingredients (redistilled) are these:

'Sphinx Pink'

Newest spring shade for lips and matching fingertips!

A vividly light, bright-at-night *power-mad* pink! More sharp than sweet, more sly than shy . . . chic-est shade in 2000 Springs! Wildly flattering—wonderfully *wearable*

'Sphinx Pink': Super Lustrous R. Lustrade, and Lanolite Lipstick, matching Nail Enamel, 'Futurama' skin by Van Cleef and Arpels for new 'SPHINX DOLL' case?)

'Sphinx Eyes'

New idea in eye makeup! Madly mysterious! Egypt-inspired!

Eyes newly shaped . . elongated . . darkly outlined for depth. Languorous lids, lightened with beige, shadowed with smoky kohl. The effect? Unforgettable! (And almost *unforgivable*!)

'Sphinx Eyes' Kit: Dream Beige Accent Shadow, Misty Grey Kohl Eyeshadow, Brown Ash and Blush/Cake Eyeliner and Eyeplotter brushes. (Available separately, or in complete kit.)

curled up with a small black cat, it was promoting subtle 'Sphinx pink' lips and smoky charcoal shades for 'madly mysterious' Sphinx eyes a full year before the release of Liz's epic historical movie – mostly because the star herself had been photographed rocking Cleopatra eyes in an array of glitzy locations, accessorised with her handsome co-star.

Within the alchemy of the Cleopatra look, there's more than a little of Elizabeth's own personality. 'I did it myself,' she once shrugged of her iconic blue-black eyes. '[Makeup artist] Alberto de Rossi prepared the sketches, but his back went out before filming began. I had studied his techniques, so I copied what I had seen him do.' Women around the world followed her lead. Decades on, there are several options for modern girls wishing to capture a little of her mesmerising Nile-side glam. Even if you're not looking to recreate the full Cleopatra, elements of the style remain hugely wearable, adding a dash of mystique to your everyday look.

1. Start with a base of very pale or off-white foundation and powder.
2. Prep your lids and below your brows with primer, such as Shadow Insurance by Two Faced. Liz's violet eyes were the focal point for this look so you'll want to paint yours in shades that last all night long.
3. Next, apply your eye shadow with a heavy hand. Although Liz wore striking Nile blue for the film – painting from her lash lines up to her brows in blocks of colour – sixties Cleopatras typically

opted for thick, white eyelids. For an updated alternative, dust your eyelids and creases with a bold peacock shade (Urban Decay's Deep End is pretty close to Liz's signature colour and imbued with multi-dimensional sheen), blending up to the brow bone with a softer, golden colour. Midnight Cowgirl, also by Urban Decay, should add a subtle finish, reminiscent of Queen Cleo's penchant for everything that glitters.

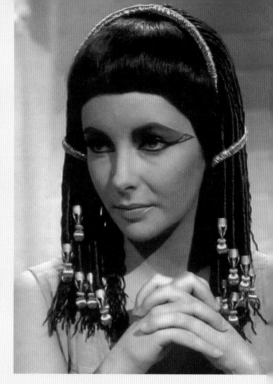

Elizabeth Taylor.

4. Apply black liquid liner generously along your upper lash lines, beginning slightly below the tear duct. Repeat the process under the eye, again starting just below the tear duct and angling the line back up towards the corner of the eye. The idea is to create Queen Cleo's angular diamond shape.

5. **Winging it! The options:** For a more wearable daytime look continue your liner beyond the outer corner of the eye, sweeping the top line upwards and the lower line downwards to create a striking 'fish-tail' effect. Highlight the space between with white eye pencil. For the full-on queenly glamour (as shown above in Elizabeth's on-screen look), extend your top line beyond the lashes, angling slightly upwards so that it's almost level with the outer edge of your brow. Repeat with the lower line, but keeping it slightly straighter so that the space between your two lines increases the further out you get. Continue a fraction further than where your top line finishes. Draw a third diagonal line to connect them in a broad, bold wing. Next, take a broader gel eyeliner pen (or a gel liner and brush if you prefer) to colour in the shape. You can use the pen to build chunkier lines around the outer corners of your eyelids if you wish.

6. Elizabeth was born with two sets of dark lashes (to the endless confusion of the crew of *Lassie* – who ordered thirteen-year-old Liz

to scrub the excess mascara off of her eyes, without realising that she was wearing none), but you can get her intriguing look with fakes.

7. Brows should be thick and angular. You can pluck your brows in straighter lines than you normally would, but it's also worth adding black eyebrow pencil to exaggerate the effect – creating striking new angles and filling out your brows.
8. Apply lipstick in a strong, bold red.
9. Finish with talon-like, blood-red nails – use fakes if necessary.
10. For true Egyptian glamour, accessorise with long, dangling earrings, an armful of bracelets, a wrap dress and, of course, the famous Sphinx Hairdo.

AUDREY HEPBURN'S MOD MAKEUP

'There is something magic about a beautifully made dress . . . you can wear it season after season with a confident feeling of being well dressed. That applies to makeup too.'

– Audrey Hepburn

With a little help from her friend Givenchy, Audrey Hepburn transformed herself into the '60s most delectable Mod icon. Her makeup in *How to Steal a Million*, created by longstanding friend Alberto de Rossi, is a perfect example of this style. Audrey's hair for the film was designed by celebrity stylist Alexandre of Paris, but maintained during filming by Alberto's wife, Grazia.

1. Apply foundation and powder to match your colouring, with just a hint of blush.
2. Follow the lash line with liquid liner, extending just beyond the corner of the eye for an exaggerated almond shape.
3. Still using your liquid liner, draw along the curve of your crease. Don't quite meet the lash line at either corner of your eye. Wait for

your liner to dry – so as not to smudge your handiwork – and then use a brush to soften the line.

4. Next, dust on a generous covering of eye shadow in a delicate pastel shade (pale yellow or baby pink would be perfect). Extend the colour to fill the shape you created with your eyeliner – take care not to go beyond the lines. For added sheen in the evening, top with cream shadow in a metallic shade.

5. Apply mascara liberally to the top and bottom lashes. Audrey herself used cake mascara for a clump-free look, but modern volumising mascara works even better. Apply a double layer to the outer lashes to give them an outward sweep. You may wish to amp them up with fake lashes, but only apply these to the outer half of your eyelids (top and bottom).

6. Finish with baby pink lipstick – in true sixties style.

7. Pluck the eyebrows only slightly, so that they are straighter and thicker closest to the nose, tapering off towards the outer edge of the eye (in line with your eyeliner). If you do pencil your brows, use a natural-looking colour.

Audrey's hairstyle was christened the 'Coupe Infante '66'. Worn short in front and longer at the back – where it was teased into a fabulous sixties-style bouffant – Audrey's stylish new hair formed the perfect frame for her beautifully made-up eyes.

BRIGITTE BARDOT'S KITTENISH VIBE

'There's no harder work than trying to look beautiful since eight in the morning until midnight.'
– Brigitte Bardot

Sex kitten Brigitte Bardot is as famous for her iconic makeup as she is for her gingham bikini. The focal points of Brigitte's look are her strikingly sultry 'cat's eyes', balanced with a pillowy nude lip.

Audrey Hepburn.

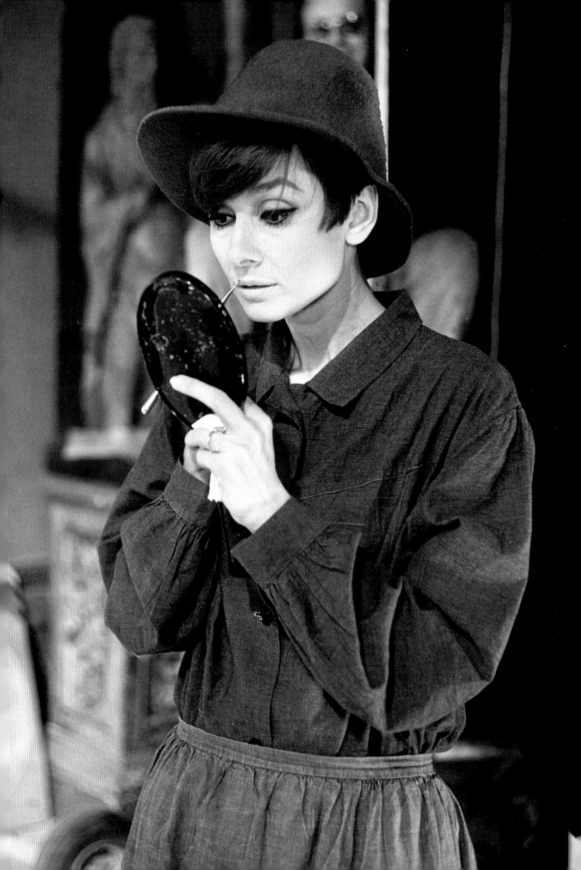

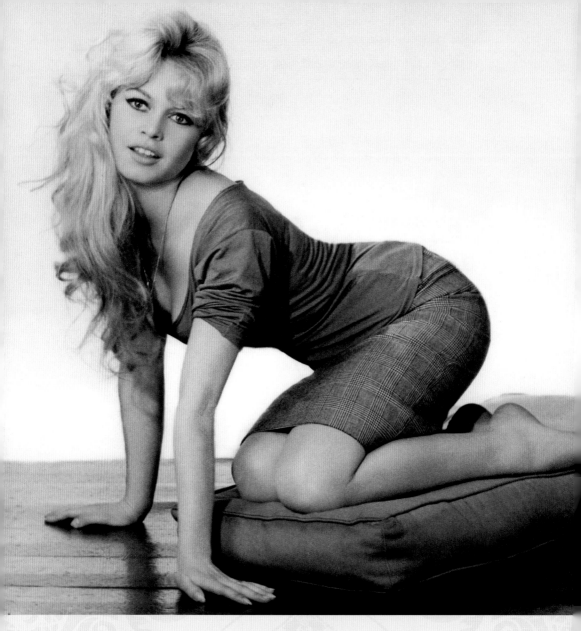

Brigitte Bardot.

Like many sixties girls, Brigitte also painted her lips with a range of pastel shades, from lime green to lavender. Slow to take off in more conservative America, Brigitte's lipsticks were shocking, young and custom-made by Parisian house, Charles of the Ritz. Designed to coordinate with her outfit, these colours were rumoured to be laced with a secret ingredient that made them 'glow' in whichever shade Brigitte happened to be wearing. Topped with sexily dishevelled bangs and

I-don't-care hair, Brigitte's winged eyes are as on-trend now as ever and have been channelled by everyone from Kate Moss to It Girls of the moment Georgia May Jagger and Suki Waterhouse.

1. If 'God Created Woman', then Brigitte certainly created the resort of St Tropez. To get her sun-kissed summer glow, apply a light covering of warm matte foundation that's not too far from your own skin tone. Brigitte's skin was often tanned, but seldom dewy.
2. Brows should be worn *au naturel*, with minimal tidying up from below. If you're not a natural blonde, you can define them with just a dusting of beige-brown eye shadow.
3. Next, prep your lids with a combination of primer and your neutral beige eye shadow of choice.
4. For added va-va-voom, brush your lids with daring black eye shadow (Nars' glitter-laden Night Breed makes for a stunning evening look). Begin at the lash line, blending up to create a subtle winged shape at the outer edges. Highlight below your brows for maximum impact. Be sure to blend.
5. To build Brigitte's dramatic winged eyeliner, you'll need a black gel liner and specialist eyeliner brush. Bobbi Brown's Ultra Fine Eyeliner brush is a perfect tool for this look, with a pointed shape that'll allow you to create BB-esque contours. Use it to draw a fine line from the tear duct, curving along the upper lashes and finish in an up-sweep at the outer corner of your eye.
6. Go back and paint over the line to build it up. The line should be thickest in the middle, tapering off at either end.
7. Repeat the process along the lower lash line. Don't worry too much if it smudges – this will only add a certain *je ne sais quoi*!
8. Apply lashings of mascara to the upper lashes.
9. To get Brigitte's bombshell pout, pencil round your natural lip lines with your peachy pastel product of choice. Fill in the shape with a matte-finish lipstick in a slightly lighter shade. If you're looking to complement your healthy summer complexion, apricot, peach and beige are your best friends.
10. Finish with a dusting of rouge – warm peachy tones on the apples of your cheeks will give you Brigitte's natural glow – and powder to set your look.
11. For the full BB impact, tease your hair into a beehive – or 'choucroute' as Brigitte would have called it.

Hair

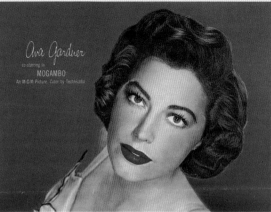

Ava Gardner
co-starring in
MOGAMBO
An M-G-M Picture. Color by Technicolor

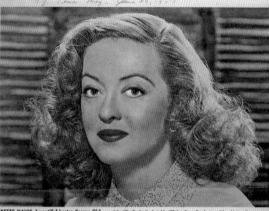

YES, AVA GARDNER uses Lustre-Creme Shampoo. In fact, in a mere two years, Lustre-Creme has become the shampoo of the majority of top Hollywood stars! When America's most glamorous women use Lustre-Creme Shampoo, shouldn't it be *your* choice above all others, too?

BETTE DAVIS, beautiful Lustre-Creme Girl, one of the "Top-Twelve," selected by "Modern Screen" and a jury of famed hair stylists as having the world's loveliest hair. Bette Davis uses Lustre-Creme Shampoo to care for her glamorous hair.

For the Most Beautiful Hair in the World
4 out of 5 Top Hollywood Stars
use Lustre-Creme Shampoo

The Most Beautiful Hair in the World IS KEPT AT ITS LOVELIEST
WITH Lustre-Creme Shampoo

Glamour-made-easy! Never was hair care easier or more rewarding. Even in the hardest water, Lustre-Creme shampoo foams into lavish, deep-cleansing lather that actually "shines" as it cleans . . . leaves your hair soft and fragrant, gleaming-bright.

Will not dry hair! Wonderful Lustre-Creme doesn't dry or dull your hair—even if you want to shampoo every day! Lustre-Creme is blessed with Natural Lanolin to make up for loss of protective oils . . . bring out glorious sheen and sparkling highlights in your hair.

Makes hair eager to curl! Now you can "do things" with your hair—right after you wash it! Lustre-Creme Shampoo helps make hair a joy to manage. Even flyaway locks respond to the lightest touch of brush or comb. And this, without any special after-rinse!

. . . and thrilling news for users of liquid shampoo! Lustre-Creme Shampoo, now available also in new Lotion Form, 30¢ to $1.00.

When Bette Davis says . . . "I use Lustre-Creme Shampoo" . . . you're listening to a great motion picture artist whose beautiful hair is part of the charm that enchants millions.

In a recent issue of the magazine, "Modern Screen," a committee of famed hair stylists named Bette Davis, lovely Lustre-Creme Girl, as one of 12 women having the most beautiful hair in the world.

You, too, will notice a glorious difference in your hair from the magic of Lustre-Creme Shampoo. Under the spell of its lanolin-blessed lather, your hair shines, behaves, is eager to curl. Hair dulled by soap abuse . . . dusty with dandruff . . . now is fragrantly clean. Rebel hair . . . is tamed to respond to the lightest brush touch. Hair robbed of natural sheen now glows with renewed sunbright highlights. All this, even in the hardest water, with no need for a special after-rinse.

No other cream shampoo in all the world is as popular as Lustre-Creme. It the best buy good for your hair? For hair that behaves like the angels, and shines like the stars . . . ask for Lustre-Creme, the world's finest shampoo, chosen for "the most beautiful hair in the world"!

The beauty-blend cream shampoo with LANOLIN. Jars or tubes, 27¢ to $2.

FAMOUS HOLLYWOOD STARS use LUSTRE-CREME SHAMPOO for GLAMOROUS HAIR

ELIZABETH TAYLOR, co-starring in Metro-Goldwyn-Mayer's "IVANHOE"—Color by Technicolor

LORETTA YOUNG, star of the forthcoming "MAGIC LADY"—A Universal-International Picture.

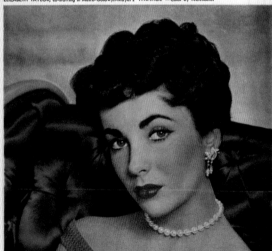

ELIZABETH TAYLOR . . . Lustre-Creme presents one of 12 women voted by "Modern Screen" and a jury of famed hair stylists as having the world's loveliest hair. Elizabeth Taylor uses Lustre-Creme Shampoo to care for her glamorous hair.

LORETTA YOUNG . . . Lustre-Creme presents one of Hollywood's most glamorous stars. Like the majority of top Hollywood stars, Miss Young uses Lustre-Creme Shampoo to care for her beautiful hair.

The Most Beautiful Hair in the World
is kept at its loveliest . . . with Lustre-Creme Shampoo

The Most Beautiful Hair in the World
is kept at its loveliest . . . with Lustre-Creme Shampoo

Yes, Elizabeth Taylor uses Lustre-Creme Shampoo to keep her hair always alluring. The care of her beautiful hair is vital to her glamour-career.

You, too, like Elizabeth Taylor, will notice a glorious difference in your hair after a Lustre-Creme shampoo. Under the spell of its lanolin-blessed lather, your hair shines, behaves, is eager to curl. Hair dulled by soap abuse . . . dusty with dandruff, now is fragrantly clean. Hair robbed of its natural sheen now glows with renewed highlights. Lathers lavishly in hardest water . . . needs no special after-rinse.

No other cream shampoo in all the world is as popular as Lustre-Creme. For hair that behaves like the angels and shines like the stars . . . ask for Lustre-Creme Shampoo.

The beauty-blend cream shampoo with LANOLIN. Jars or tubes, 27¢ to $2.

Famous Hollywood Stars use Lustre-Creme Shampoo for Glamorous Hair

When Loretta Young says, "I use Lustre-Creme Shampoo," you're listening to a girl whose beautiful hair plays a vital part in a fabulous glamour-career.

You, too, like Loretta Young, will notice a glorious difference in your hair after a Lustre-Creme shampoo. Under the spell of its lanolin-blessed lather, your hair shines, behaves, is eager to curl. Hair dulled by soap abuse . . . dusty with dandruff, now is fragrantly clean. Hair robbed of its natural sheen now glows with renewed highlights. Lathers lavishly in hardest water . . . needs no special after-rinse.

No other cream shampoo in all the world is as popular as Lustre-Creme. For hair that behaves like the angels and shines like the stars . . . ask for Lustre-Creme Shampoo.

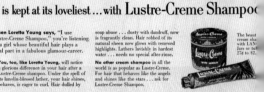

The beauty cream shampoo with LANOLIN. Jars or tubes, 27¢ to $2.

Hair Care

'I think that the most important thing a woman can have, next to her talent, is her hairdresser.'
– Joan Crawford

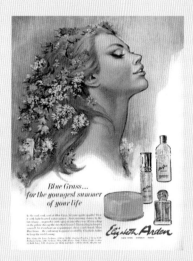

Blue Grass...
for the youngest summer
of your life

Elizabeth Arden

As much as your signature scent or the cut of your LBD, it pays to pay attention to your tresses. 'In Hollywood, a girl's virtue is much less important than her hairdo,' Marilyn once stated. And she wasn't wrong. Meticulously styled to fit their public personas, actresses' hair had everything to do with how they were perceived by directors, their co-stars and the world. Famed for her cascading curls, it was only after Mary Pickford dared to bob her hair that she was able to grace the screen as a woman rather than a little girl. Likewise, redheaded Rita Hayworth made a career of playing fiery femmes – until husband Orson Welles decided to cast her in his film noir, *The Lady From Shanghai*. This slippery, shady role marked the reinvention of Rita as an ice-cool blonde. In short, any starlet who wished to stay in the spotlight, with room to grow and develop, had best be prepared to make daring updates to her signature style, or else find one that worked for her and stick with it, in the style of the inimitable Lauren Bacall.

For modern girls, hair is no less crucial a concern. It can be your crowning glory, glowing with personality and styled in harmony with your features, or an unmanageable, day-ruining mess. Here's how to make every hair day a good day, vintage-style.

'A dowdy, untidy hairdress is bad enough in everyday life, but on the screen it simply isn't tolerated.'
– Ginger Rogers

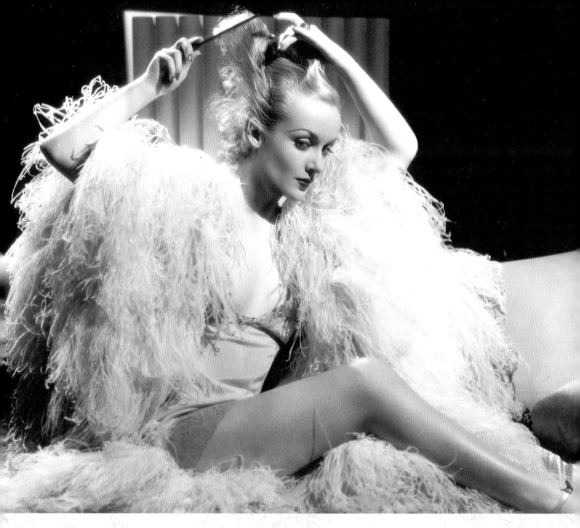

Carole Lombard.

BRUSHING

'If you brush it every night, I don't think you'll ever have any serious hair problems.'
– *Vivien Leigh*

- Brush bristles should be 'sturdy enough to penetrate the underneath layers of hair, yet flexible enough so that they will not scratch the scalp,' advises *Hollywood* beauty editor, Ann Vernon. This provides a healthy massage for the scalp and stimulates circulation.

- For increased shine, Janet Leigh recommends all-natural bristles.
- 'Hair should always be brushed away from the scalp and never flat down,' advises Helen Turpin, head stylist at 20th Century Fox in the sixties: so bend over and get brushing, ladies!
- 'Don't think because it's naturally curly you can't brush it,' says Max Factor. Regular brushing increases the vitality of the hair, so even curls need attention.
- 'Be sure to keep your brush clean . . . giving it a bath in mild soapsuds and warm water at least once a week,' says Ann Vernon.

DRY-CLEANING YOUR HAIR

Perfect for mornings when you pressed the snooze button once too often, this simple vintage tip can help you refresh lank, greasy locks even if you don't have time to shower. Back when frequent washes (any more than once a week) were believed to be bad for your hair, Hollywood's leading ladies gave themselves regular dry-cleans with Turkish (terry-cloth) towels, massaging vigorously down to their roots for bouncy, cleaner-looking locks.

VERONICA LAKE'S HOME HAIR TREATMENTS

'I would have preferred to have made my mark with a shorter hairstyle. Everything would have been easier.'
– Veronica Lake

- Double brush! Veronica plied one natural bristle brush in each hand.
- Ten-minute head massages, rubbing with the tips of her fingers.
- Butter-rub treatment. The night before a drying shampoo, Veronica

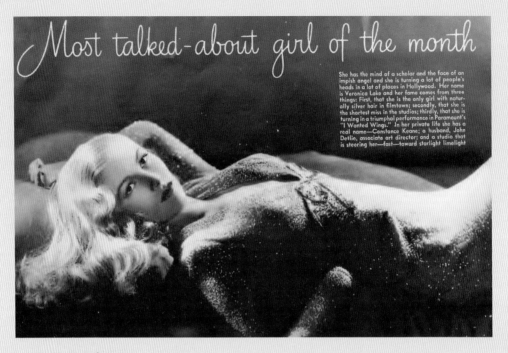

She has the mind of a scholar and the face of an impish angel and she is turning a lot of people's heads in a lot of places in Hollywood. Her name is Veronica Lake and her fame comes from three things: First, that she is the only girl with naturally silver hair in filmtown; secondly, that she is the shortest miss in the studios; thirdly, that she is turning in a triumphal performance in Paramount's "I Wanted Wings." In her private life she has a real name—Constance Keane; a husband, John Detlie, associate art director; and a studio that is steering her—fast—toward starlight limelight

Veronica Lake.

would apply a tablespoonful of melted butter to her scalp with a cotton cloth. According to Veronica, the salt in the butter acts as a stimulant, helping the butter to be absorbed. Finally, she'd wrap her hair in an old towel and retire for her forty winks.

- Lemon conditioner, containing 4ml of freshly squeezed, strained lemon juice and 120ml of warm water. After shampooing, Veronica would douse her hair with this mixture. As well as conditioning, the juice acted as a natural bleach, keeping Veronica's colour vibrant. Just don't forget to rinse out if you're not blonde.

TIPS FOR COLOURED HAIR

'I said I wouldn't dye anymore, unless they wanted me to be bald for the rest of my life.'
– Lana Turner

By the mid-forties, over sixty percent of actresses were rocking coloured locks (according to Max Factor, Jr). Thankfully, these bottle-blonde (and redhead and brunette) beauties developed their own ways to combat the frizz.

JEAN HARLOW

'Castor oil not only prevents dryness,
but it gives a beautiful lustre to the hair.
Anyone who has seen me will tell you, I think,
that my hair really does have a sheen.'
– Jean Harlow

Jean swore she never dyed her hair . . . but her platinum locks did require 'treating' every other day to keep them looking, well, *platinum*. Jean's treatment of choice was a combination of 'white soap' (Lux flakes), peroxide and 'French bluing' (a tint often seen on the hair of elderly ladies, this helped prevent her platinum shade from turning yellow). To keep this toxic combination from destroying her hair too thoroughly, Jean's tips were brushing for softness, Castile-soap shampoo and that vintage standby, castor oil. Rather than add further chemicals, she set her waves with water and vinegar.

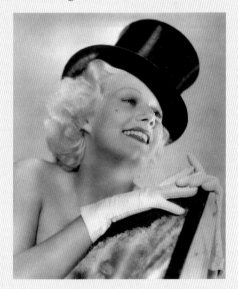

Jean's castor-oil rub – to be used before every colour treatment:
- Heat up some castor oil, but 'make sure it's the odourless kind,' Jean warns.

- Rub the oil well into the roots of your hair and leave for several hours.
- Wash out the oil to reveal beautiful locks.

How to make Jean's Castile-soap shampoo:
- Grate an average-sized bar of Castile soap (or any vegetable oil-based soap) into five cups of water.
- Boil until all the soap is dissolved and then cool.
- Store in a jar until it is required.

GINGER ROGERS

'If you think your hair is a nuisance,
think of us poor stars, who have to allow
about one hour a day for our hair!'
– Ginger Rogers

Although Ginger is synonymous with beautiful auburn locks, she changed her colour often. Her favourite shades were coppery red and platinum blonde. Thankfully, Ginger's mother also knew a home remedy for damaged hair: pure coconut-oil, rubbed into the scalp once a week (ideally the night before shampooing). Ginger herself had one more indispensible tip. 'Sunshine gives life to your hair,' she once said. 'It strengthens the scalp. It gives the scalp a tingling, warm feeling . . . and wakes up your mind, too.' So, why not treat your hair to fifteen glorious minutes a day?

RITA HAYWORTH

'Everyone knows that the most
beautiful thing about Rita was her hair.'
– Harry Cohn, President of Columbia Pictures

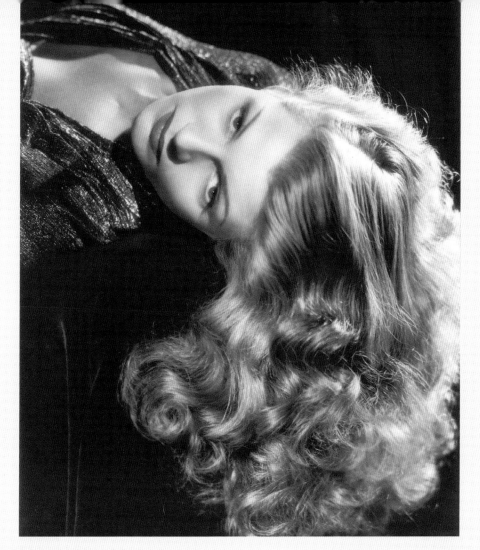

Rita Hayworth.

America's redheaded sweetheart liked a few days' dark growth to frame her face, but she still needed to dye her hair every week and shampoo every four days. Here are Rita's tips for keeping your hair sleek, manageable and glowing:

- After shampooing, saturate your hair with olive oil and wrap in a towel for fifteen minutes. Rinse with hot water and lemon juice to remove the grease.
- To prevent split ends, always comb your hair in sections.
- For really bad hair days, use a final rinse of one part white vinegar and nine parts lukewarm water. It makes hair easier to handle and 'gives it a glint'.

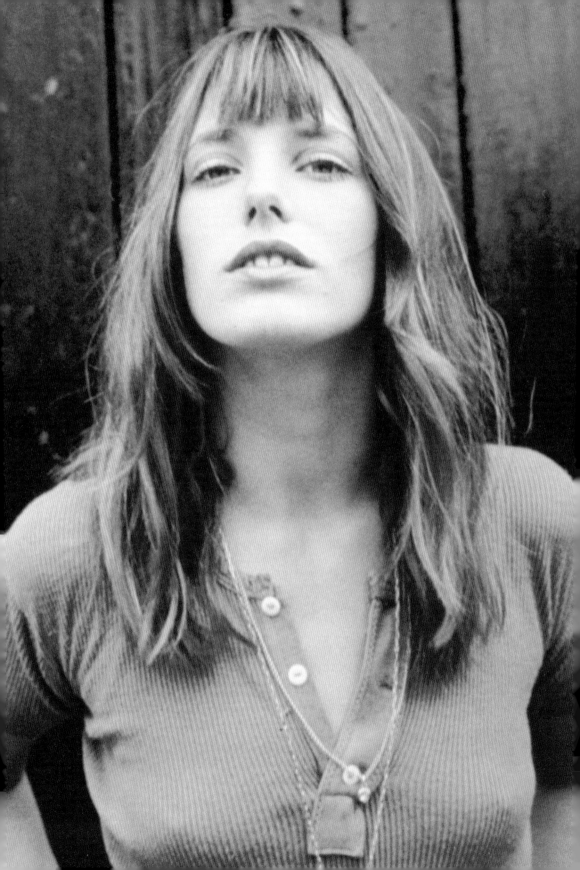

Styling to Suit Your Shape

*'A good hairdo projects confidence
in a woman and changes her personality.'*
– Alexandre of Paris, celebrity hairdresser

As transformative as rouge, highlighter or foundation, you can use your hair to disguise or enhance, spotlight or soften your facial features. Here's a selection of corrective cuts and instant fixes that you can discuss with your stylist, helping you to trim your way to ovalescent perfection!

HIGH FOREHEAD (OBLONG).
Bangs are your best friend.
Your hairspiration: Alexa Chung. Brit It girl of the moment Alexa has always possessed an eye for wearable vintage styles. Inspired by effortless '60s beauties Jane Birkin and Jean Shrimpton, her tousled bangs help to shorten and soften her classic oblong shape.

NARROW/LOW FOREHEAD (TRIANGLE).
Soft curls and waves can help add width across your temples. Fluffed-up bangs – à la Katharine Hepburn in *Little Women* – will also help balance out your shape. If in doubt, sweep it back and wear it high!

Your hairspiration: forties dream girl Rita Hayworth. Rita's cloud of tumbling curls, swept over in an adorable side-parting, is perfect for any girl wishing to broaden out her forehead. Punk princess Kelly

Jane Birkin.

Osbourne is often glimpsed wearing a lavender version of Rita's ultra-feminine style.

BROAD FACE (SQUARE).

Experiment with off-centre partings – in this way you can create soft curves to frame your face, whilst offsetting the angles of your jawline nicely.

Your hairspiration: Veronica Lake's cool, asymmetric waves – featuring a side-part that curves high over the crown of her head and *that* sultry peek-a-boo curl – are an ideal solution for any girl looking to slim down her cheeks.

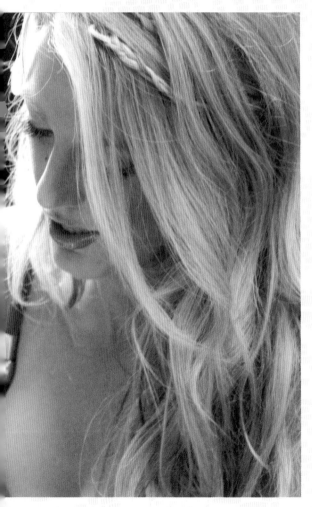

PROMINENT JAWLINE (SQUARE).

Use gentle curls and beach waves to mask the angles of your jaw, whether this means embracing your natural texture or reaching for the barrel curling iron. Rather than tucking hair behind your ears, allow it to fall naturally. Ladies with square jawlines should wear their curls lower on their necks. Avoid cuts that stop at your chin; these will only *add* width to your jaw.

Your hairspiration: To create her tousled tresses (reminiscent of the bed-headed waves worn by Brigitte Bardot in the '60s), Blake Lively – queen of twenty-first-century bohemian cool – prefers to 'air dry'. 'I leave it three percent wet and sometimes put the tiniest bit of mousse in it,' she revealed. 'Then I put it up in a ballerina bun. It gives it a little more bounce so it doesn't dry flat. My hair has a slight natural wave to it, so it will hold that.'

Blake Lively.

POINTED CHIN (INVERTED TRIANGLE).

Flatter your delicate jawline with choppy layers and/or bouncy curls that fall to just below your cheekbones. The added volume should balance out your features. Ladies with natural widow's peaks, rising up in a heart shape, should wear them with pride!

Your hairspiration: Marilyn Monroe's loose-and-lovely curls showcase her widow's peak to perfection. Her fellow starlet Dorothy Dandridge – the first ever African-American to be nominated for an Academy Award – wore her gorgeous afro curls in a similar face-framing style, proving that Marilyn's windswept bob suits all manner of textures.

LONG FACE (OBLONG).

Add width to your face with waves and curls. Since it's only the length of your face that needs balancing out, you can rock a centre-parting like no other face shape.

Your hairspiration: Liv Tyler. Best known for her cameo as an elvish maiden in the *Lord of the Rings* trilogy, Liv's locks are no less beautiful in real-life. Though she's experimented with various looks throughout her career (including a pixie crop circa 1998, that seemed far too severe for her elegant, elongated features; 'My hair was down to my waist until the amazing stylist John Sahag cut off my ponytail,' remembers Liv), long-faced Liv will always be synonymous with glossy chestnut waves, channelling the timeless red-carpet glamour of Lauren Bacall et al.

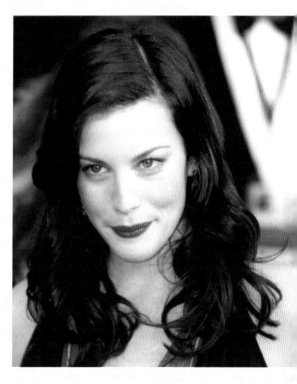

Liv Tyler.

LARGE FEATURES.

A full-on lioness or bouffant bob will make your striking features appear more delicate, without altogether drowning them out.

Your hairspiration: Brigitte Bardot, Farrah Fawcett, Julia Roberts, Beyoncé Knowles – none of these beauties are afraid of big, bold hair and

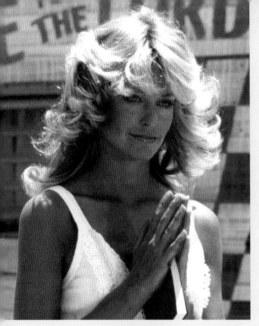

Farrah Fawcett.

neither should you be. And if you're naturally curly, be sure to embrace your wild side with diffuser-dryers and volumising product.

DELICATE FEATURES.

Short and sweet crops – sixties pixies or smooth, close-fitting bobs – will showcase your gorgeous bone structure.

Your hairspiration: Audrey Hepburn, Mia Farrow, Mary Quant and Nancy Kwan. In the fifties and sixties, each of these long-haired beauties opted to go for cutting-edge crops with stunning results. Decades on, the pixie crop is still the last word in short and oh-so-sweet chic, rocked by such celebrities as Emma Watson, Anne Hathaway and Michelle Williams.

EXTREME STYLING

Not content with sweeping hair back to lengthen the face, Hollywood took this principle to the extreme, with many leading ladies subjecting themselves to electrolysis in the quest for the perfectly defined hairline. Rita Hayworth had hers raised one whole inch by this expensive, excruciating treatment. 'They took photos of Rita,' explained her stylist Helen Hunt, 'blew them up and drew lines indicating where the hairline should be. The change was important, but subtle. I used to bleach the front of Rita's hair, so the hairline wouldn't be so prominent – the cameramen were always after me to lighten her hair.'

Many other stars, including Marilyn Monroe and Jayne Mansfield, had 'alterations' made. Lucille Ball, however, was one actress who refused to have her hairline raised. 'That's a great big project,' said the sensible star, 'and I have no intentions of becoming a slave to it'. Yet another reason to love Lucy . . .

Rita Hayworth.

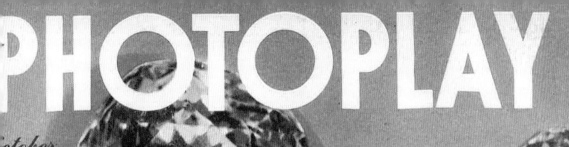

PHOTOPLAY

October

15c

t Pictures

ll Color of

Hayworth's

neymoon

ayworth

al Hesse

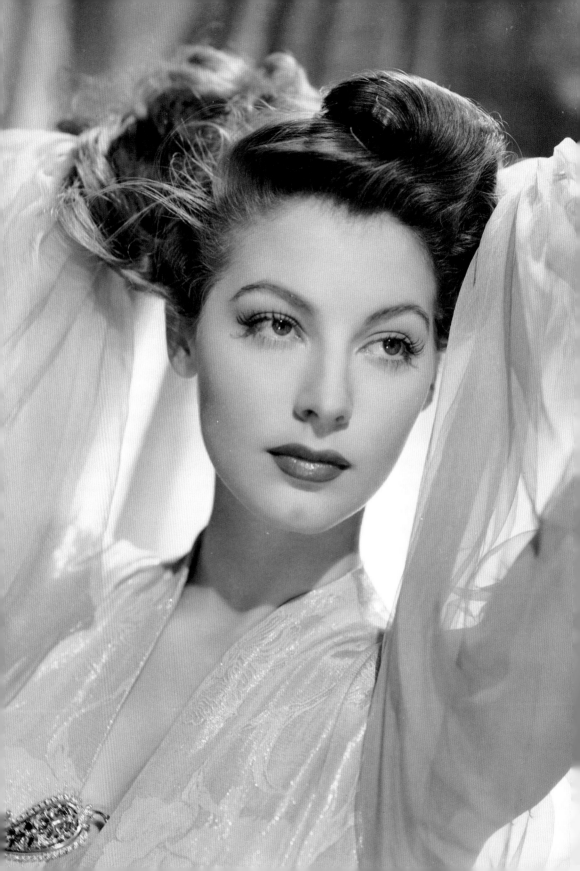

Vintage Styling: The Basics

YOUR ESSENTIAL STYLING KIT

- Natural bristle brush
- Bobby pins – to secure your pin curls, curlers and to hold up chignons and rolls
- Wave pins – long double-pronged, spring-set pins for securing finger waves, rolls and stand-up curls
- Grip-Tuth hair combs – to secure rolls, pin back waves or attach flowers and ribbons
- Rat-tail combs – for sectioning up hair, tucking the ends into pin curls and rolls and teasing those bouffants
- Rollers – preferably made from perforated plastic to let the air through. Hot rollers will give you more structured curls, faster
- Pin curlers – a substitute for your fingers, use these nifty little sticks to roll up your hair, then slide a bobby pin in to keep them in place
- Hair net (or a scarf) to keep your pin curls in place whilst you sleep
- Ribbons
- Wave set (true vintage vixens may wish to experiment with a sugar-water solution)
- Barrel curling iron (since the marcel iron is no longer available to buy)
- Cats, rats, mice and switches – to raise your beehives and rolls to new heights without the backcombing
- Hairspray – it's the only way to keep that bouffant up!

Ava Gardner.

MAKING WAVES

MARCEL WAVES

Created by the curling iron of Parisian coiffeur François Marcel in the 1870s, these natural-looking waves caused a sensation in '20s Hollywood. Designed to follow the contours of the head, marcel waves look fabulous when added to a neat bob and many more styles

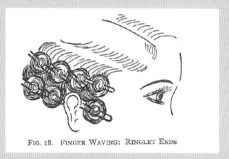

FIG. 18. FINGER WAVING: RINGLET ENDS

besides. Jean Harlow's undulating waves, ending in a profusion of fluffy pin curls, are an example of marcelling at its best. Modern-day curling irons make it easy to recreate this look at home. Starting at the root, curl sections of hair under, then over to create Marcel's trademark S-shape. Secure with wave pins to set your style.

FINGER WAVES

For a less sculpted look that's not so long lasting, opt for finger waves. Begin styling whilst your hair's still wet, shaping into waves with a tail comb. Secure with wave pins and leave to set (beer, sugar water and chemical wave were once the styling products *du jour*). Used to

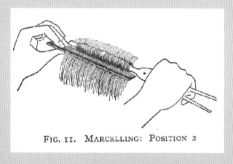

FIG. 11. MARCELLING: POSITION 2

add gorgeous texture to twenties bobs, they can also be incorporated into longer styles. Joan Crawford's look, for instance, combines finger waves with pin curls.

CURLS

'Bob pins, remember, are utilitarian not ornamental!
That is my statement for the day.'
– *Ann Vernon*, Hollywood *magazine*

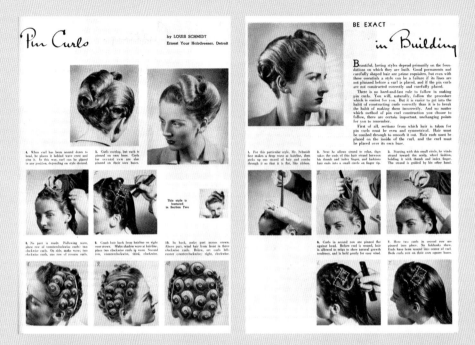

PIN CURLS

An incredibly versatile style, pin curls can be tight or loose, combined with waves or even poker-straight locks. Many thirties girls would wear just a small line of pin curls along their hairline, brushed out to create the famously fluffy bangs sported by Katharine Hepburn in *Little Women*. In the 1940s, curled bangs became a real style statement with great mops of curls being worn up front. All-over curls made a comeback in the fifties when Lucille Ball's 'poodle' style was all the rage.

Pin-curl rules:
- The less hair you use, the tighter the curl.
- Hair must be curled inward so that the end of the hair lies within the curl.
- The curl must always be pinned over its own base.

STAND-UP CURLS

Also known as barrel curls, these rolls of hair are pinned to the head upright and are useful for making bigger, wider curls (think Marilyn Monroe). They're especially good if your hair's not quite long enough to go around a roller.

Maureen O'Hara's tips for managing naturally curly hair:
- Wash your hair. While it's still wet, pull hair straight and roll into large pin curls.
- Sit under a dryer until it's *almost* dry.
- Brush hair out into a loose wave.

'Before I came to Hollywood and learned this trick, I couldn't do a thing with my hair,' says Maureen.

ROLLERS

Pencils, strips of fabric and folded paper . . . anything that you can wrap your hair around constitutes a roller. Today's rollers are plastic and perforated for quicker-drying curls. For making waves or adding volume to the bouffant styles of the late fifties and sixties, they're a vintage essential.

Left: *Loretta Young*. Right: *Ingrid Bergman*.

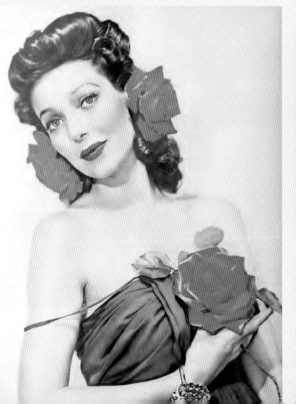
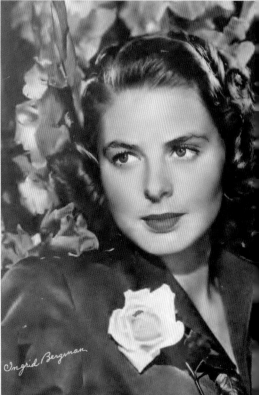

Tips for roller girls:

- To create loose, soft curls, wrap large sections of slightly damp hair round each of your curlers.
- For smaller, tighter curls, apply extra water and wind less hair.
- Always opt for perforated curlers – they allow the hair to dry faster.
- The bigger the roller, the bigger the volume.
- Make sure hair is *really* dry before taking out the curlers. While you're waiting, simply don a headscarf or 'donna cap' (a forties-style hairnet with a chin strap) and leave over night. Alternatively, speed things up with a hairdryer.

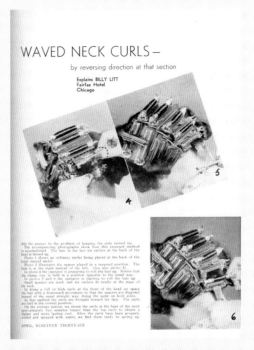

ROLLS

'The days of straight expanses of hair are gone. The smartest coiffures feature waves, curls and rolls.'

– Ann Vernon, Hollywood magazine

Forties girls began styling their hair in flirtatious rolls of all varieties. The last word in utilitarian chic – there's no prettier way to keep hair out of your eyes – rolls can be achieved by winding sections of hair around your fingers (ideally backcombed and prepped with hairspray beforehand), rolling them up and pinning them to the top or the side of your head. Types of roll – as rocked onscreen by Ava Gardner, Rita Hayworth, Betty Grable and co. – include:

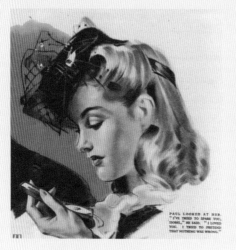 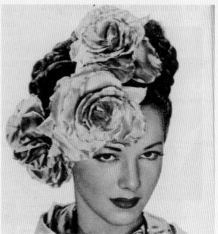

- Single rolls – set at an angle to create a simple, striking look.
- Angel rolls – hair is centrally parted and each half rolled tightly in at the side of the head to create a look like angels' wings.
- Victory rolls – named after the daredevil manoeuvres of bomber pilots, victory rolls are the last word in wartime chic. Perfect for hard-working factory girls and modelled by Veronica Lake, this government-approved style entails two large rolls at the front with hair at the back curled up and away from the nape of the neck in a kind of 'reverse pageboy'.
- Roll bangs – a pin-up style made famous by Bettie Page, roll bangs are not really rolls at all; they're pin curls. The setting is exactly the same as for fluffy bangs (another pin-up favourite), but instead of brushing the hair up from underneath, hair is smoothed over towards the brow.

BACKCOMBING

Essential for all sixties bouffants, backcombing involves holding sections of hair up at right angles from the head and 'teasing' it down towards the roots with a fine-toothed comb. It's not great for your hair, but it does add instant volume.

FINISHING TOUCHES
– ACCESSORIES WITH ATTITUDE

'So great is the interest in hair ornaments that no girl dares show her head in the evening any more without a flower or clip decorating her topknot.'

– Hollywood *magazine*

Fabulous flappers take note: a '20s bob demands a jewelled barrette or decorative band.

'I never worry about diets,' Mae West once quipped. 'The only carats that interest me are the number you get in a diamond.' Blonde bombshells should make these their words to live by, adorning their locks with all that glitters.

For a look that lasts one night only, accessorise with natural blossoms. Joan Crawford found flowers 'more fragrant and easily matchable' with her gowns than any precious stone, whilst Greta Garbo layered on the exotic mysticism with delicate white orchids.

Chanteuse Grace Moore (aka the Tennessee Nightingale) playfully teamed her gowns with flocks of tiny, feathered songbirds.

As rocked by Bette Davis and Claudette Colbert in the 1930s, pin-on braids are perfect for girls wishing to flirt with longer styles without the up-keep. Wear them straight across, at a jaunty angle, curled in a classy coronet or customised with ribbons.

Functional ribbons, turbans and headscarves remain *de rigueur* for all would-be forties pin-ups hoping to bag themselves a sweetheart in the forces. For a perfectly co-ordinated look, try making them out of off-cut material from your dress.

To capture the spirit of the flirty '50s, wrap your ribbon around a swinging high ponytail à la Audrey Hepburn in *Sabrina*. Team with a matching scarf on days when you're feeling impossibly cute.

Top your voluminous Bardot beehive with a chunky black bandeau and copious amounts of attitude.

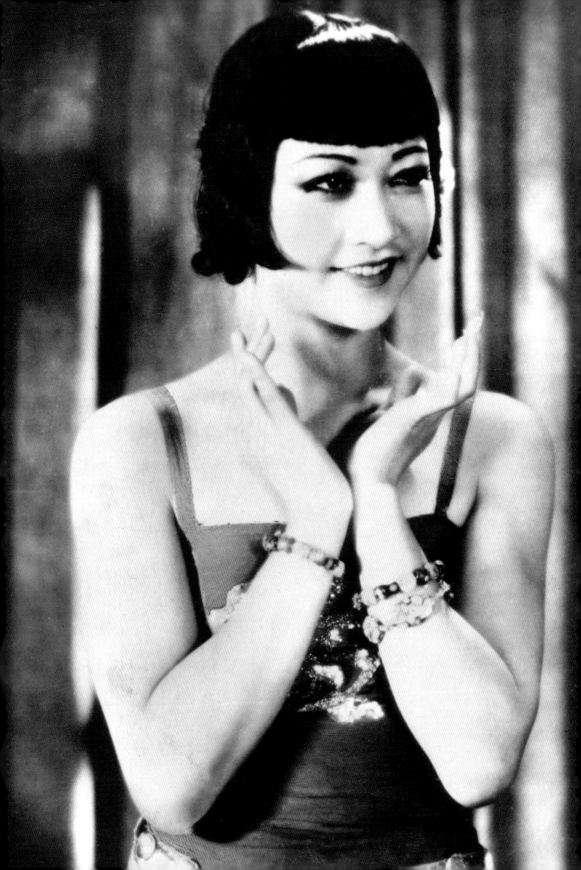

Making Headlines: The Best Vintage Crops

THE LOUISE BROOKS BOB

'I might as well confess my secret: I'm a cliptomaniac!
Cutting hair amounts to an obsession with me . . . I find
short hair very convenient for every type of coiffure.'
– Gloria Swanson

Whether you wore yours curly or shingled, windswept or slicked back, bobbed hair was all the rage in the 1920s. A dramatic change from the long locks fashionable up until this point, the bob was fun, edgy and refreshingly low-maintenance. Perhaps the most iconic variant of all is Louise Brooks' Dutch bob. Created by

Anna May Wong.

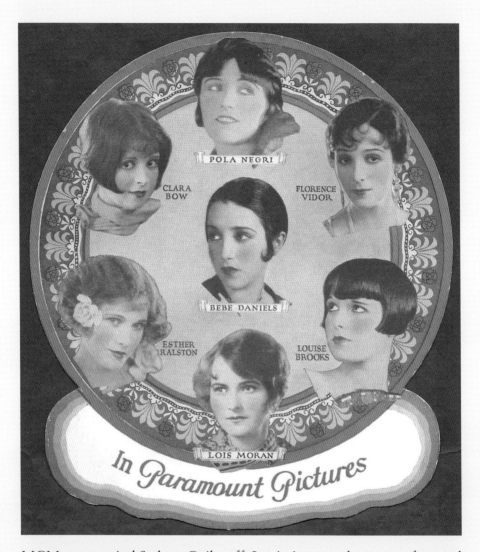

POLA NEGRI

CLARA BOW

FLORENCE VIDOR

BEBE DANIELS

ESTHER RALSTON

LOUISE BROOKS

LOIS MORAN

In Paramount Pictures

MGM mastermind Sydney Guilaroff, Louise's razor-sharp crop featured a severe centre-parting and heavy, straight-cut bangs. Not relieved by so much as a finger wave, this daring cut was the polar opposite of the cascading curls popularised by girl's girls Mary Pickford and Lillian Gish, and embraced by fearless flappers everywhere.

Though curly girls can still rock this look (if you're prepared for the extra upkeep), it is tailor-made for hair with a naturally smooth, straight texture, as demonstrated by trailblazing beauty Anna May Wong, the very first Chinese-American siren in Hollywood. As much as the bob flattered her gorgeous bone structure, Anna May revealed that chopping off her locks 'took a lot of thought. A Chinese woman's hair is her chief ornament in life, so we could not possibly approve of bobbed hair. Some Chinese women think it is dangerous to the femininity and beauty of a woman!' Thankfully, Anna May was not one of them.

1940S PAGEBOY BOBS

'They don't take so much living up to as uppish,
more elaborate coiffures.'

– Vivien Leigh

In the 1930s and '40s, bobs grew longer and more feminine, adding versatility to the charms of the original cut. Hair could be rolled under for a practical daytime look with the option to add curls, braids and ornaments for dazzling evening glamour. Inspired by the curled-under boy cuts glimpsed in many a medieval romance, pageboy hair should be between shoulder and chin-length, and cut into a curved shape that's shortest around the face and longer at the back. To get the classic pageboy, set your hair in rollers (or stand-up curls) to add volume and to iron out any natural kinks. Be sure to roll under rather than over. Once your curls are set, you can begin brushing them out till they're pageboy-smooth. Brush on the underside of the hair, rotating your brush as you go for a perfect 'curled-under' look.

Smoky-voiced siren Lauren Bacall rocked her own customised version

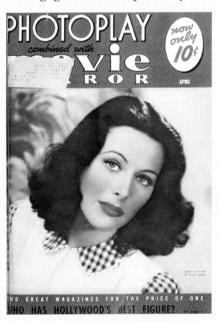

PHOTOPLAY *combined with* **Movie MIRROR** *now only* 10¢ APRIL

TWO GREAT MAGAZINES FOR THE PRICE OF ONE

WHO HAS HOLLYWOOD'S BEST FIGURE?

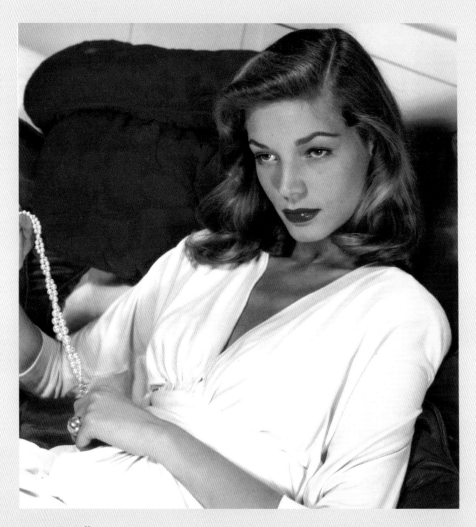

Lauren Bacall.

of the pageboy throughout her starry career and beyond. In Lauren's own words, 'the wave on the right side, starting to curve at the corner of my eyebrow and sloping downward at my cheekbone' was not something she was prepared to modify for anyone. Sticking with her lustrous, face-framing waves was clearly the right choice; the first time husband Humphrey Bogart ever kissed her, she was seated in her trailer combing them out. Here's how you can achieve her touchably soft look at home. In true Lauren-esque style, wear with one side swept up and fastened in place with a comb or a slide.

THE VERONICA LAKE PEEK-A-BOO

'It just falls naturally that way now,
even just after I wash it.'
– Veronica Lake

Really just an extra-long version of the forties bob, the addition of a single pin curl, drooping luxuriantly over one eye, was enough to transform Veronica's hair from enviable to iconic. The story goes that Ms Lake was mid-screen test when a stray lock fell over her eye; the studio loved it and decided to make her a star! Whatever the truth, the look became wildly popular; so much so that the US government was forced to ask Veronica to change it during the war. Too many girls, filling men's jobs in factories, were risking their lives for Veronica's vision-impairing waves. Veronica did the patriotic thing and rolled up her trademark locks. Accidents fell by twenty-two percent. She also participated in a series of public service films where she posed with her beautiful hair trapped in machinery . . .

Veronica Lake.

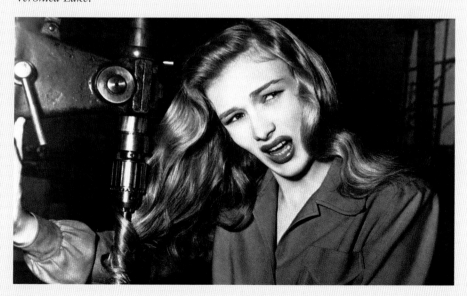

Indeed, Veronica herself found the peek-a-boo frustrating. In real life, it got caught in buttons, jewellery and – once, apparently – an elevator door. A chain smoker, Veronica also set her hair on fire on a fairly regular basis. When she wasn't filming, she preferred to wrap her locks up in a turban or braids – two chic, practical styles that were very popular at the time. After the war, Veronica hoped to keep the use of both her eyes but the studio wouldn't allow it; the peek-a-boo was written into her contract.

Peek-a-boo stats:
- Veronica's hair measured twenty-four inches at the back; seventeen at the front.
- Her hair hung straight for six inches and then fell in waves.
- With the exception of *that* pin curl, Veronica's waves were natural.
- The style droops over the eye through sheer weight of hair, thanks to the deep side parting.

THE SCARLETT O'HARA

Created by MGM hair genius Sydney Guilaroff, Vivien Leigh's Georgian belle style in *Gone with the Wind* kicked off one of the forties' hottest hair trends. Known as the half-up, half-down, the style is created with two rolls – one on each side of the head – secured with combs. The back of the hair hangs loose in a long bob, or gathered in a hairnet. You'll see subtle variations on this style. But whether it entails a mop of many curls à la pin-up supreme Betty Grable, or two large ones, all these half-up 'dos lead back to Vivien Leigh's unforgettable turn as the headstrong Scarlett.

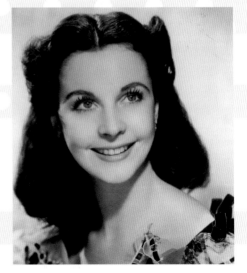

Vivien Leigh.

THE POMPADOUR

Inspired by Louis XV's mistress, Madame de Pompadour, and a staple of '40s pin-up girls, the pompadour is really just an extra-large roll on the top of the head.

Tips for a basic pompadour:
- Divide the front half of the hair into three sections, so that you have one low side-parting on each side of the head.
- Next, brush the central section up and away from the head. It should then be rolled back and pinned to the crown of the head with bobby pins.
- The sides are often brushed back and secured with a clip, or more bobby pins decorated with a ribbon or flowers.

As the pompadour only really refers to the front of the hair, you can do almost anything you like with the back. Seen here, Rita's hair has been pin-curled beforehand, adding to the height of the pompadour. Larger versions of the pompadour can be made by brushing the hair over a 'rat' (or its smaller relation, the 'mouse'). Pinning back the sides will increase the impact of this style and is particularly effective if you have stunning features like Rita's. Pair with bright red lips and a can-do attitude! For the full Rita Hayworth look, this style looks fabulous peeking out of a snood.

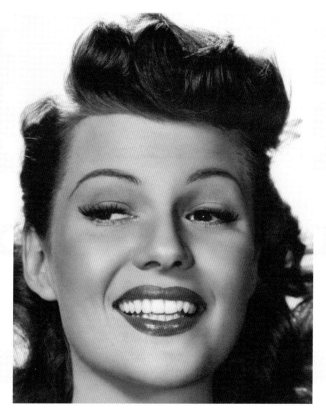

Rita Hayworth.

GRACE KELLY'S SUPER CHIGNONS

Inspired by the looks created by Alexandre of Paris in the fifties, the **low chignon** was one of Grace's favourite casual looks. Her hair was usually kept in a long bob, making it an ideal length for this simple style. Here's how you can recreate her timeless chic:

1. Make a low ponytail and secure with a clip or ribbon.
2. Roll hair around two fingers then, slipping the fingers out of the roll, fold the hair inwards towards the nape of the neck until you create a flat 'pear' shape.
3. Secure the roll with bobby pins, just below your ribbon.

Grace's look was always very neat, but this style also looks good with a few straggling hairs to frame it. Pair with a silk scarf tied jauntily around your neck and simple, natural makeup.

For more formal occasions, Grace often favoured a **banana chignon**. For this sleek and stylish look, it's best to roll or straighten the hair before you start. Once you've ironed out any natural kinks:

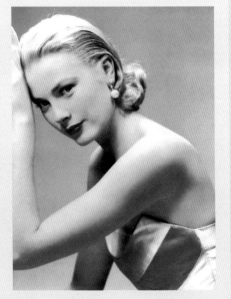

Grace Kelly.

1. Brush hair into a low ponytail.
2. Twist the ponytail once and lift up so that it lies flat against your head.
3. Holding the hair reasonably taut, roll your ponytail in on itself and secure with pins.
4. Team with a pearl necklace and simple hair ornaments.

MARILYN MONROE'S
WINDSWEPT CURLS

With its choppy layers, loose curls and platinum hue, Marilyn's bob is one of the most iconic styles of all time. She created it with large stand-up curls, brushed back from the brow and left in partial disarray to create a relaxed, windswept look.

Although Marilyn's platinum curls inspired millions of imitators from Italy to India, by 1950s standards, her hair was actually something of a mess. Incredibly, Marilyn topped a number of 'worst coiffed' lists, with beauty experts referring readers to the more refined styles of Grace Kelly or Claudette Colbert. But what it lacks in 'good grooming', Marilyn's style more than makes up for in fuss-free, youthful charm. It's still one of the most copied styles of all time – and deservedly so. These days, all you need to become a twenty-first-century bombshell is a chunky barrel curling iron.

Top tip! Subtle changes can keep your favourite look feeling fresh. Look closely and you'll realise that Marilyn never wore her hair *exactly* the same for any two movies and her shade of blonde varied from diamond (almost white) to champagne (with a yellow tint).

THE AUDREY HEPBURN CROP

'What used to be the Italian boy hairdo is now more frequently described as a "Hepburn-type" crop.'
– *Cynthia Lowry*, Associated Press

The trend for boyish cuts started in Italian cinema, but it took Audrey Hepburn's transformation from princess to pixie in 1953's *Roman Holiday* to inspire women everywhere to chop off their locks. Short crops soon became hugely popular in Hollywood and beyond, varying in length from four inches to one. Many of the styles, like the 'bubble' and 'Greek god' cuts, incorporated tight curls. Though various Hollywood starlets experimented with boyish cuts, you need very delicate features to pull off this style. Elizabeth Taylor made it work for her for a while, but Lana Turner quickly found her glamour was in her hair.

'Audrey is the most intriguingly childish, adult, feminine tomboy I've ever photographed.'

– Celebrity photographer, Mark Shaw

Of course, Audrey has always been queen of the pixie cuts. She sported a number of crops over the years – some curling around her ears and the back of her head (see *Roman Holiday*), others much shorter, like the choppier cut she wore when she picked up her Oscar for the same film. Whatever the overall effect, Audrey almost always opted for short bangs, highlighting her incredible, statement eyebrows. Women didn't just want Audrey's hair; they were enamoured of her entire look. Tellingly, sales of ballet slippers in the US soared to one and a half million pairs the year that Audrey appeared in *Sabrina*.

ELIZABETH TAYLOR'S SULTRY SPHINX

Made famous by Elizabeth Taylor in the epic historical movie, *Cleopatra*, this style was invented by Alexandre of Paris, and evolved into a slightly more wearable evening style, courtesy of Elizabeth Arden.

Alexandre's Parisian sphinx. Hair is cut in two layers. The top layer is teased into a bouffant with straight-and-severe bangs across the forehead. The second layer entails a chin-length bob, poker-straight, but curling under at the edges. Ideally, your extravagant earrings should dangle just below the hair line.

'Add a ponytail for effect, slather black liner on your eyes, part two eyeliners at the sides and you're an American version of the Egyptian Queen.'

– Myrna O'Dell, Miami News

Elizabeth Arden's American sphinx. For ladies who were not so lucky as to be able to book an appointment with the famous Alexandre, Elizabeth Arden created a more easy-to-maintain alternative. This version kept the bangs, but gave them a slight wave, softening the effect. Hair was bouffant at the front but left slightly longer at the back and often worn in a ponytail.

THE HOLLY GOLIGHTLY

Audrey Hepburn always had her finger on fashion's pulse and, with a little help from her friend Givenchy, she completely reinvented her style for the 1960s. If Audrey set a trend with the pixie cut she wore in *Roman Holiday*, it was nothing to the sensation she would create with her Holly Golightly up-do a decade later.

One of cinema's most iconic styles, Audrey's hair in *Breakfast at Tiffany's* is bouffant at the front with the back rolled into a high chignon and streaked with caramel-blonde highlights. Hair streaks first became fashionable in the 1950s (Alexandre of Paris also takes credit for this trend), but Audrey took them to new heights (literally) in the classic movie. Like most sixties hair trends, these streaks were intended to make an impact, rather than imitating natural highlights. Of course, the ever classy Audrey manages to make them look chic, not cheap.

Audrey Hepburn.

THE BARDOT BEEHIVE

A variation on the bouffant is the massive sixties beehive made famous by Brigitte Bardot, created with lots of backcombing and even more hairspray. Here are the basics:

1. Using a rat-tail comb, divide the hair into three-inch-wide sections, starting at the crown.
2. Tease each section of the hair back towards the root – starting from about two inches from the crown.

Brigitte Bardot.

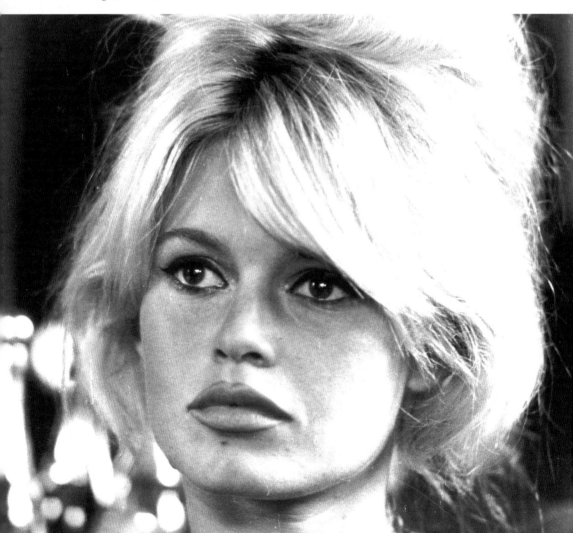

3. Give each section a good spray and then smooth hair gently back over the resulting hornet's nest. The 'bump' on the crown of your head should be the focus for this style.
4. Either leave hair hanging loose, tie with a ribbon, or sweep up and secure with bobby pins.
5. For a true Bardot look, leave your hair deliberately dishevelled. Pair with a headscarf, lots of winged eyeliner and a heavy tan.

SIXTIES SHORTS AND THE NANCY KWAN

'Nancy Kwan's bob was the shot that put me on the map . . . it motivated a whole new feeling.'

– Vidal Sassoon

These neat crops may seem completely unrelated to the long, bed-headed styles worn by Bardot and co., but they were the start of the rebellion against 'artificial' beauty and hours spent in the salon. The sixties also marked the revival of the bob, accompanying a fresh wave of youth culture, shorter hemlines and new freedoms. As in the twenties, bobs were cut close to the nape of the neck to emphasise the shape of the head. They were designed to be 'fuss-free' – allowing sixties girls to just wash, brush and go. After all, this generation had better things to do than sit in a salon all day!

Vidal Sassoon gets most of the credit for bringing bobs back into fashion; his 'five-point cut' on Grace Coddington – though the model turned editor now insists, 'he didn't create it for me; he created it on me' – caused an instant sensation. But it was the simple, asymmetric style he created for 'Chinese Bardot' Nancy Kwan in 1963 that really launched Sassoon as a star stylist. Nancy wore the cut in the film, *The Wild Affair* and the 'Nancy Kwan' quickly became one of the most requested styles of the early sixties. The style was tailor-made for Kwan and clearly looks fantastic on her. Yet, even if you don't possess her sleek, black locks, don't despair. According to Sassoon, the beauty of this shape is that it suits almost every face shape and hair texture. As the decade went on, bobs got shorter so that they were barely longer than so-called 'boy crops', another major sixties trend.

BEST OF THE BOY CUTS

Jean Seberg. Jean's extreme boy cut works only on the most beautiful and delicate of faces. Jean first cut her hair to play Joan of Arc – the powerful female lead – in her very first film, *Saint Joan*. Yet, it was her subsequent roles in *Bonjour tristesse* and *À bout de souffle* that would make the boy cut her signature style. Naturally pixie-like, Jean seemed born to wear this style.

Mia Farrow. Although she was far from the first actress to go for the chop, Mia Farrow's super-short boy cut shocked audiences and created a genuine sensation. Although publicity photos show Vidal Sassoon hovering over Mia with the shears, Mia actually cut her own hair using ordinary nail scissors. An already-famous Sassoon trimmed off an extra half-inch for the cameras (and was paid $5,000 for doing so). Mia made the look more striking by wearing almost no makeup, which added to her fragile, childlike charm. For a true Farrow look, pair with shift dresses and coloured tights.

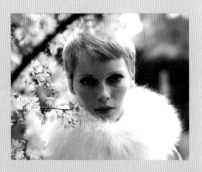

Mia Farrow.

Crop tips:
Only go for this cut if you have delicate features and an oval, round or heart-shaped face.
Remember: short hair exposes the neckline. Keep yours looking as pretty as your face with moisturising creams and, if necessary, body makeup.
Short hair is a great excuse for chic neckwear: accessorise with necklaces, little scarves or Peter Pan collars.

THE 1960S BOUFFANT BOB

The opposite end of the spectrum from the minimalist Nancy Kwan was the bouffant bob, a high-impact hairdo popularised by the likes of Jackie Kennedy. The style was created with extra-large rollers and lots of hairspray – the bigger the roller, the higher the hair. In the salon, a bouffant meant hours beneath the dryer; at home, it meant a sleepless night in rollers so big you couldn't lie down. Despite the discomfort you had to go through to obtain it, the bouffant was so popular that it is now one of the most recognisable styles of the sixties.

A bouffant bob doesn't really need further embellishment, so finishing touches were usually quite simple. Jackie rolled the ends of her hair, either out or under; while Jane Fonda opted to set hers in large pin curls. Accessories – perhaps a plain headband or ribbon – were equally understated, keeping the spotlight on the bouffant itself.

For a quick bouffant look straight from the 1960s, *Hairdo* magazine recommended this cheater's method:

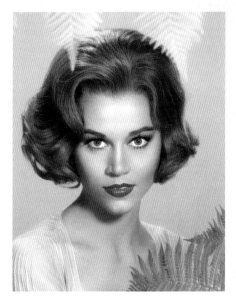

Jane Fonda.

1. Set rollers in dry hair around the top of the head and cheeks, then spritz just the rollered sections with hairspray.

2. Leave the hairspray to dry – this should take between fifteen and twenty minutes – then start brushing the hair out gently.

3. About halfway through your comb-out, blast the whole head with hairspray before continuing to brush. Then spray again.

4. Fix the details with a rat-tail comb while the spray's still damp.

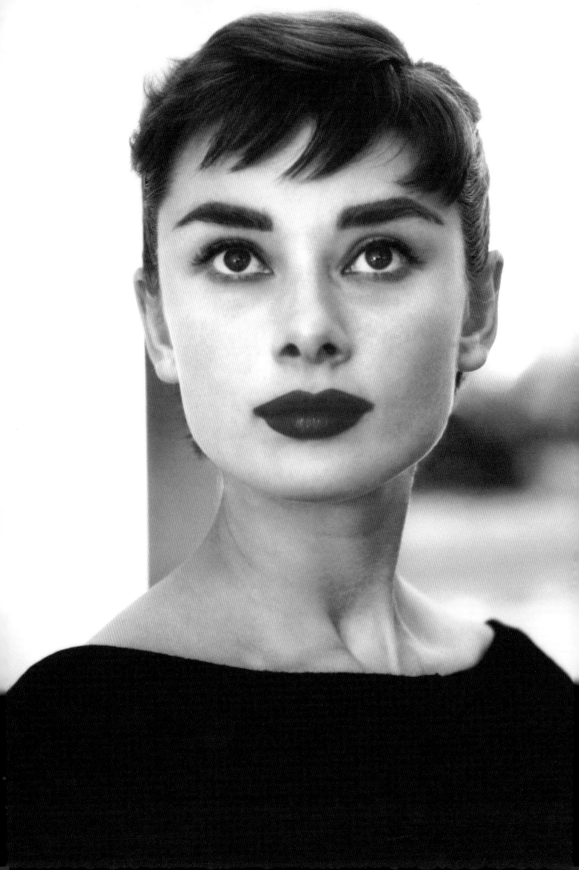

Conclusion:
Beauty and
Individuality

*'Above all else, insist upon your
right to be an individual.'*
– Carole Lombard

One day, Veronica Lake was walking through a hotel lobby when she spotted a woman sporting her own trademark peek-a-boo hair. The woman shot Veronica a look of pity; she didn't recognise the star who had wisely discarded the hazardous one-eyed look off-screen. Veronica simply smiled. 'I know you,' she thought to herself. 'You're a dime Veronica Lake.'

This is the best lesson we can learn from Hollywood's most beautiful stars: no carbon copy is ever as good as the original. A Veronica Lake look-alike is only ever a Veronica Lake look-alike. Marilyn Monroe might have dyed her hair platinum blonde to match her idol Jean Harlow, but she became an icon by developing a style all of her own. Bette Davis longed for Katharine Hepburn's striking features – 'those gorgeous, beautiful cheekbones! What a face' – but soon learned to appreciate the features she was born with. 'Not having as definite a face, I could wear any kind of hair or makeup and always look like a different person,' she said. That versatility helped Bette escape the

Audrey Hepburn.

typecasting of the Hollywood star system and show all that she had to offer as an actress.

The secret to true beauty is creating a look that is particular to you. Ava Gardner, Audrey Hepburn, Brigitte Bardot, Marilyn Monroe, Sophia Loren all made a mark on popular culture that is very much their own. 'They possess very individual beauty,' said makeup artist Alberto de Rossi of the most beautiful actresses he had ever worked with. 'Joan Crawford had that type of uncopyable beauty – distinct, individual, different.'

None of these women had a perfect face – well, except perhaps Ava Gardner – but Joan Crawford made wide lips desirable; uneven teeth gave charm to Audrey Hepburn's twinkly grin. Sophia Loren's feline

Carole Lombard.

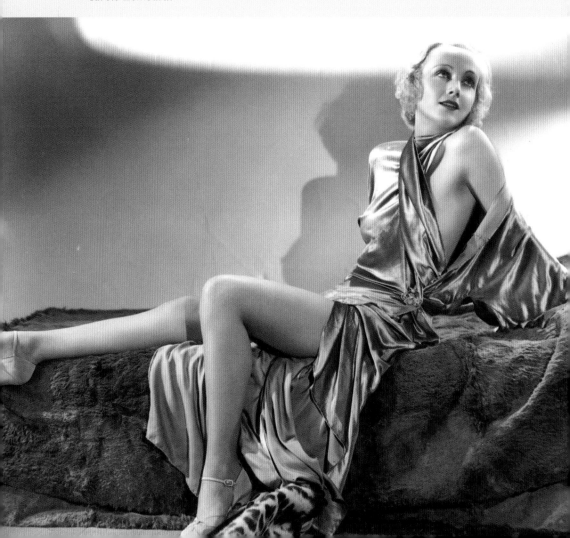

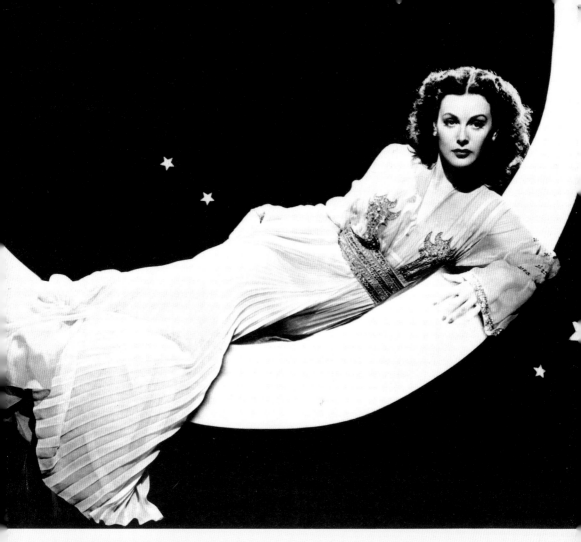

Hedy Lamarr.

eye makeup was designed to play up her very best feature and Brigitte Bardot's voluminous tresses made an impact her pretty face alone could not have achieved. As Joan Crawford herself says, 'most women can counterfeit beauty'; it's just a question of playing to your strengths.

Looking to the past for inspiration allows us to escape modern trends and create a look that is one-off – that's what vintage style is all about. The key is to find your style – and then to learn to love it. 'The girl who is forever primping, who is eternally outlining two perfect bow-lips, or whose hair is lacquered into place – that girl is not beautiful – she is uncomfortable,' said exotic beauty Hedy Lamarr, revealing perhaps the best beauty secret of all: self-acceptance. None of us are without flaws, but the truly beautiful woman is happy in her own skin.

Published by Plexus Publishing Limited
The Studio, Hillgate Place
18-20 Balham Hill
London SW12 9ER
www.plexusbooks.com

ISBN-13: 978-0-85965-508-8

Cover photos by Getty Images/Bettman;
Getty Images/John Kobal Foundation;
Getty Images/Bettman; Getty Images/Keystone/Stringer
Cover and book design by Coco Balderrama
Printed in Great Britain by Bell & Bain Ltd.

Bibliography
Books: *Greta Garbo: A Life Apart*, Karen Swenson;
Garbo, Barry Paris; *Notorious: The Life of Ingrid
Bergman*, Donald Spoto; *Ingrid: A Personal Biography*,
Charlotte Chandler; *Ava Gardner: Love is Nothing*,
Lee Server; *Hollywood Goes Shopping*, David Desser;
Hollywood and the Rise of Physical Culture, Heather
Addison; *How to be Lovely: The Audrey Hepburn
Way of Life*, Melissa Hellstern; *Marlene Dietrich's
ABC*, Marlene Dietrich; *Pull Yourself Together, Baby*,
Sylvia Ullback; *Hollywood Undressed: Observations of
Sylvia As Noted by Her Secretary*, Sylvia Ullback; *No
More Alibis*, Sylvia Ullback; *The Science of Beautistry*,
Marinello; *Beauty Book*, Polly Bergen; *A Film Star's
Way To Glamour*, Ann Hastings; *Hollywood Hairstyles*,
Arlene Dahl; *Encyclopaedia of Hair: A Cultural History*,
Victoria Sherrow; *How To Be Adored: A Girl's Guide to
Hollywood Glamour*, Caroline Cox.
　　Magazines and Newspapers: *The Pittsburgh Press,
The Pittsburgh Post-Gazette, The Spokane Daily
Chronicle, The Lakeland Ledger, The Ocala Star
Banner, The Palm Beach Post, The Spokesman Review,
The Reading Eagle (PA), The Milwaukee Journal, The
Milwaukee Sentinel, The St Petersburg Times (FL), The
Toledo Blade, The Miami News, The Miami Sunday
News, The Nashua Telegraph, The Schenectady Gazette,
The Montreal Gazette, Sarasota Herald-Tribune, The
Deseret News, TV Radio Mirror, The Spartanburg
Herald Journal, The Palm Beach Morning Post, The
Eugene Register-Guard, The Kentucky New Era, The
Ottawa Citizen, The San Jose News, The San Jose
Evening News, The Sunday Independent (FL), The Day,
The Dispatch (NC), The Lakeland Ledger, The Kingman
Daily Miner, Albany NY Knickerbocker News, The
Florence Times Daily (AL), The Diamondback (MD),
The Lodi News Sentinel, The Wilmington Star News,
The New Straits Times, The Prescott Evening Courier,
The Florence Times Daily, The Lewiston Daily Sun, The
Berkeley Daily Gazette, The Melbourne Age, The St*

*Maurice Valley Chronicle, The Coaticook Observer, The
Sydney Morning Herald, The Independent, The Chicago
Daily Tribune, The Boston Globe, The Los Angeles
Times, Photoplay, Life, Hollywood* magazine, *Coronet*
magazine, *Click, Motion Picture Magazine, Picture Play*
magazine, *American Hairdresser* magazine,
Hairdo magazine.
　　Journals: 'World War II and Fashion: The Birth of
the New Look,' Lauren Olds, *Constructing the Past:*
2001; 2:47-64; '"Speak softly and Carry a Lipstick":
Government Influence on Female Sexuality though
Cosmetics During WWII,' Adrienne Niederriter,
Deliberations: 2010, 11: 4-9.
　　Websites: www.1920-30.com, www.cosmeticsandskin.
com, www.besamecosmetics.com, oldmagazinearticles.
com, Redbookmag.com, beautyhigh.com, atomicredhead.
com, glamourdaze.com, vintagemakeupguide.com,
dailymail.co.uk, glamourmagazine.co.uk, instyle.co.uk,
vogue.com regissalons.com, www.marvingwestmore.
wordpress.com, www.nickyclarke.com, www.elle.
com, www.stylist.co.uk, fashion.telegraph.co.uk, www.
huffingtonpost.com, www.theglamourologist.blogspot.
co.uk, www.loti.com, www.gildedslippervintagestyle.
blogspot.co.uk, www.dirtylooks.com, www.hrc.utexas.
edu/exhibitions/web/gwtw, www.seraphicpress.com/
veronica-lake-goes-to-war.
　　We would like to thank the following for images:
Weegee (Arthur Fellig)/International Center of
Photography/Getty Images; Duke University Library
Collection; Woodbury/Duke University Library
Collection; Helga Esteb/Shutterstock.com; Movie Market;
General Photographic Agency/Stringer/Getty Images;
Bourgeois/Duke University Library Collection; Helena
Rubenstein/Duke University Library Collection; Chris
Jackson/Staff/Getty Images; Keystone-France/Getty
Images; Lux soap/Duke University Library Collection;
Glamourdaze/Duke University Library Collection;
Hulton Archive/Stringer/Getty Images; Savage/Duke
University Library Collection; Revlon; Elizabeth Arden/
Duke University Library Collection; Dolce & Gabbana;
Yardley/Duke University Library Collection; Keystone
Pictures/Stringer/Getty Images; Hollywood Magazine/
Duke University Library Collection; Savage; Maybelline/
Duke University Library Collection; Polly Bergen's Beauty
Book; Loic Venance/Staff/Getty Images; Duragloss/Duke
University Library Collection; Cutex/Duke University
Library Collection; Revlon/Duke University Library
Collection; Photoplay/Duke University Library Collection;
Guerlain/Duke University Library Collection; Michael
Ochs Archives/Stringer/Getty Images; Popperfoto/
Contributor/Getty Images; Maybelline/Glamourdaze/
Duke University Library Collection; Everett Collection/
Shutterstock.com; Hollywood Magazine/Duke University
Library Collection; John Kobal Foundation/Contributor/
Getty Images; Terry O'Neill/Contributor/Getty Images;
Ullstein Bild/Contributor/Getty Images; Lustre – Crème
Shampoo/Duke University Library Collection; Paramount
Pictures/Plexus Archive; Eric Carpenter/Contributor/
Getty Images; American Hairdresser Magazine/Duke
University Library Collection; Everywoman Magazine/
Duke University Library Collection; Print Collector/
Contributor/Getty Images; Gamma/Plexus Archive; Kobal
Collection/Plexus Archive; Bettman/Contributor/Getty
Images; Keystone Features/Stringer/Getty Images.